Equine Herbs & Healing

An Earth Lodge Pocket Guide to
Holistic Horse Wellness

Equine Herbs & Healing

An Earth Lodge Pocket Guide to Holistic Horse Wellness

By Maya Cointreau

E. Barrie Kavasch & Sandra Cointreau

Foreword by Allen M. Schoen, MS, DVM

An Earth Lodge® Publication

Roxbury, Connecticut

*** This book contains valuable information carefully researched, but it is not intended to take the place of proper veterinary care and expertise. Please seek qualified professional care for health problems. ***

Also by Maya Cointreau:

Practical Reiki Symbol Primer

The Comprehensive Vibrational
Healing Guide

The Healing Properties of Flowers

Grounding and Clearing

The Girls Who Could Series

Equine Herbs & Healing

Natural Animal Healing

Magical Mudras

Conversations with Stones

Shamans Who Work with the Light

"A horse! A horse! My kingdom for a horse!"

~ Shakespeare

TABLE of CONTENTS

"First, you must trust in yourself.
Then you can also trust in the earth or gravity of
a situation, and because of that, you can uplift
yourself. At that point, your discipline becomes
delightful rather than being an ordeal or a great
demand. When you ride a horse, balance comes,
not from freezing your legs to the saddle, but from
learning to float with the movement of the horse
as you ride. Each step is a dance, the rider's dance
as well as the dance of the horse."
Chogyam Trungpa Rinpoche,
"Shambala: The Sacred Path of the Warrior"

FOREWORD

Herbs have been used for centuries to treat various ailments in horses throughout the world from China to Europe. Numerous folklore tales abound about horses that responded to various herbs for different conditions. The integration of these old stories and herbal formulas with conventional western veterinary medicine and healing in the 21st century is challenging.

Maya and Barrie have combined their experiences and knowledge of the traditional use of herbs with some of the latest studies in western herbal medicine. They offer an intriguing combination of scientific, practical, energetic and traditional knowledge that portrays a rational use for herbs for horses.

Controversies abound in the use of herbs with horses. Some scientists feel that the individual principle active ingredient of herbs should be isolated and their mechanism of action completely understood prior to clinical use. However, many medications have been developed and clearly state that their mechanism of action is not clearly understood. Medical and pharmaceutical researchers and clinicians believe that the active principle of plants should be identified, extracted, purified and administered in specific dosages to ensure safety. Some feel that no herb should be used without double blind placebo controlled trials. Some herbs are potentially toxic to horses. All these considerations are certainly not unreasonable in an ideal world and in an ideal situation. From the opposite perspective, often well intended individuals may suggest old folk remedies for horses that they feel have withstood the test of time as far as efficacy and safety goes. They may feel that the folklore itself is sufficient justification for use. Personally, I feel that either extreme does not do justice to our equine companions. I feel that judicious use of herbs based on the various levels of evidence available may be of benefit to horses in particular situations for both prevention and wellness as well as therapeutically where appropriate.

However, it is not uncommon that one is in a situation where conventional medications are not working or are having side effects and where surgery is not a reasonable option. In situations like this, you should search for a veterinarian that is trained in herbal medicine for horses in order to assist you in deciding whether certain herbs or formula's might be appropriate for your equine friend. There is a paucity of research on western herbs for horses, though more is becoming available. There is some research on Chinese herbal formulas for horses.

In an ideal world, there would be humanely conducted well-documented studies on all the various herbs that may be beneficial for horses. However, most research these days is conducted or supported by pharmaceutical companies which do not have any financial benefit or interest in studying herbs for horses, unless it is to develop a future medication. This is simply a matter of economics. Then we are caught in a "catch-22" where we are often cautioned to not use certain herbs that have a reasonable record of safety and efficacy unless there are current and well-documented scientific studies and yet there is insufficient funding for appropriate studies. A reasonable balance between these concerns must be addressed.

In this book the combination of knowledge on "old healing formulas" with some of the latest studies on the therapeutic and preventive use of various herbs for horses provides a great deal of useful information for both horse's caretakers and veterinarians. Maya and Barrie have combined valuable information from around the world and through the centuries along with some of the latest research on herbal therapies. Judiciously placed throughout the book are some of the most beautiful quotes about horses I have ever read, making the reading and learning process much more enjoyable and intriguing. They combine the wisdom of the ages and various cultures with the heart of their love of both horses and herbs.

This book is an informative, valuable contribution to a small but growing volume of knowledge concerning the use of herbs for horse wellness and prevention. Read, learn and enjoy as they take you through a wealth of information that may well be of great benefit to you and your kindred spirits!

Allen M. Schoen, MS, DVM, Author, "Kindred Spirits: How the Remarkable Bond Between Humans and Animals Can Change the Way We Live," www.drschoen.com

"Brahma was excessively sparing with earth, water, and fire. The new creature was not given either horns or claws, and his teeth were only meant for chewing, not for biting. The prudent care with which fire was used made him a necessity in war with out making him warlike.

This animal was the Horse.
The reckless expenditure of air and ether in his composition was amazing. And, in consequence, he perpetually struggled to outreach the wind, to outrun space itself. Other animals ran only when they had a reason, but the Horse would run for no reason whatever, as if to run out of his own skin. He had no desire to chase, or to kill, but only to fly on and on and on until he dwindled into a dot, melted into a swoon, blurred into a shadow, and vanished into vacancy.

The Creator was glad.

He had given habitations to his other creatures, forests to some, caves to others, but because of his enjoyment of the disinterested spirit of energy in the Horse, he gave him an open meadow under the eye of Heaven."
-- Rabindranath Tagore

INTRODUCTION

"A horse is worth more than riches."
~ Spanish Proverb

This book celebrates the birth of an idea spun from creative minds devoted to herbalism, horses and other animals, and healing. It is exciting to bring good minds together. The three of us have greatly enjoyed our journeys and working together. We are women warriors and business women devoted to change. We are each Reiki Masters, practitioners of energy healing, and we each bring unique and different skills to this book, and our business of Earth Lodge Horse Herbals.

All of the pathways to healing have special interests for us as well as our animals. Scientific, clinical, practical, energetic, and spiritual often work together to perfect a positive outcome. We are fortunate to be living in this age of advances in complementary medicine that welcomes all forms of healing modalities that can work together in synchronicity. Our passion for horses is something that we share with most people around the world wherever horses have a role in making life better.

Earliest Horses

"... at the very end of one gallery, where the cave floor begins a sharp drop, is a scene of high drama: a horse is falling down a rock pillar, its legs sprawled helplessly in the air."

~ Margaret Cooper (on Lascaux) in *Exploring the Ice Age,* 2001.

Peoples' earliest relationships with horses are well documented in the haunting Ice Age cave paintings in Altamira in Spain, and Lascaux and Pech-Merle in France, where horse images were created more than 20,000 years ago by our distant ancestors, the Cro-Magnons. The smooth, worn ivory of a mammoth's tusk carved into a horse some 30,000 years ago by a Cro-Magnon artist is two and a half inches long and called the Vogelherd Horse after the cave in Germany where it was discovered. Archaeologists believe the carved animal images were carried by the hunter for good luck. These are the oldest known artistic renderings, and numerous theories work to explain these mystical images of the earliest wild horses.

Horses were probably first domesticated from wild horses by central Asian nomads in the Third millennium B.C. Scientists believe these were the wild horses of Mongolia we call the Przewalski's horse today, *Equus Przewalski.* Horses were recorded in

Mesopotamia and China about 2000 B.C., Greece by about 1700 B.C., Egypt by around 1600 B.C.), and India by about 1500 B.C. Horses were domesticated in Western Europe by 1000 B.C. The term *horse* commonly refers to the modern domestic *Equus caballus,* in its many varieties.

The horse has always cast a spell on people, and continues to gallop a tantalizing line between mystery, work, pleasure, and healing. Horses and people are closely wedded in some unusual partnerships that have glittered through time. And horses are the special glue that brings this book together and binds our healing work with compassion and resolve.

In North America

Great herds of prehistoric horses and camels once grazed across the grasslands of North America during the Pleistocene

Age, but gradually became extinct by about 10,000 B.C. The next wave of horses in the Americas began when Columbus brought 24 stallions and 10 mares to the Island of Hispaniola on his second voyage for Spain in 1494. Columbus complained to King Ferdinand that he had paid for good horses, only to find that peasant horses were loaded on his ships. The antique American horse strains trace back to this hardy Colonial Spanish peasant horse brought over in narrow wooden ships: the, Garrano, Ginetes, and Sorraias varieties. The regal Andalusians came later.

More Spanish horses arrived when Spain colonized Cuba in 1511, and the first herd of cattle was brought over by Gregorio Villalobos in 1520 near Tampico, Mexico. Rugged Spanish horses acclimated well to America. These hardy equine bloodlines predate the horses brought by the Dutch, French, and English over a century later. The Spanish conscripted Indians to herd their horses, and in time Indians became skilled horsemen themselves, who escaped with some of these prized "Magic Dogs." Indians bonded with horses in many dynamic ways and evolved into the noble "Horse Cultures" of the American West, depicted and immortalized in native beadwork and artwork.

Explorers along the Appalachian Indian frontier in 1755 noted that the Chickasaw had the finest horse breed in North America, which was more intelligent and hardier than horses from England that had begun to arrive in America in about 1750. Indians had a natural talent for breeding horses.

Various Plains Indian tribes soon became famous for breeding fine horses. When Lewis and Clark crossed the Rocky Mountains in the early 1800s, they traded for horses with the Snake Indians who were well mounted on sturdy horses descended from early Spanish stock. Breathtaking reports from the 1800s document races between U. S. Calvary officers' fine horses and the smaller horses of the Comanche and Sioux Indians who beat them. Some of these escaped Indian ponies were the ancestors of the modern mustangs, the wild horses of the west.

Modern breeders believe that the few remaining Chickasaw and Cherokee horses today are our closest links to the exceptional Chickasaw horses of two centuries ago, who were the ancestors of the American Gaited breeds: the American Saddlebred Horse, the Tennessee Walking Horse, and other laterally gaited horses. Two major groups of modern horses—the light, swift southern breeds, called light horses, and the heavy, powerful northern breeds, called draft horses—are believed to have developed independently. The small breeds called ponies may derive from a southern, light horse and from a wild race. There are many valuable breeds of horses, and what was once a diverse work animal, the horse has become a chosen "pleasure animal" today.

"It is not enough for a man to know how to ride; he must know how to fall."
~ Mexican Proverb

Our Love of Horses

"Whoever said a horse was dumb, was dumb" ~ Will Rogers

We are drawn to horses in many ways, for many reasons. Throughout time horses have cropped up in human conversation as well as livelihood and art. Someone has good "horse sense" not to "horse around" with too many "horsey types." Most of us are wedded to "horsepower" and like our information straight from the "horse's mouth"; we don't "get up on a high horse" too often, we know when to "hold our horses," "rein in our desires" and we try not to "look a gift horse in the mouth!" The horse plows up an interesting 'turn of phrase' in all walks of life.

Connecticut, Massachusetts, and New Jersey have more horses per capita than other states in the United States. Connecticut has been the number one in this distinction for years; one horse for every 68 people in 2004! This is because the horse is a "pleasure animal" today bred and groomed for riding, jumping, show, and performance.

We can honestly say we live in "Horse Country" where riding trails crisscross our villages and land is set-aside in Open Space parcels where people will have more places to ride their horses. Beautiful horse farms dot the landscape and many more veterinarians today are practicing complementary medicine, especially with large animals. These environments and circumstances naturally stimulated our herbal interests in developing healing and wellness formulas for equestrian needs. It has been quite a experience to work with respected veterinarians, horses, and horse-lovers all along the way.

The Authors, in the Northwest Hills of Connecticut, 2005

"When God created the horse, he said to the magnificent creature: I have made thee as no other. All the treasures of the earth shall lie between thy eyes. Thou shall cast thy enemies between thy hooves, but thou shall carry my friends upon thy back. Thy saddle shall be the seat of prayers to me. And thou will fly without any wings, and conquer without any sword." ~ The Koran

CHAPTER ONE

A Dash of Herbalism

Hast thou given the horse strength? Hast thou

clothed his neck with thunder? ~ Job 39:19-25

Herbalism has been a practiced art among people for over 7000 years. Archaeologists have found that the first human crops consisted of over two hundred different plants, many of which were grown for their medicinal qualities. Today, indigenous people around the world still possess an arsenal of herbal knowledge which has been passed down from generation to generation for centuries.

In Ancient China, the emperor **Chin Nong** (3494 BCE) was believed to have been one of the regions' first herbal doctors, oral tradition has preserved stories of his dedication to the study of

1

new medical plants and remedies throughout his life.   Acupuncture, an Asian technique of influencing the healthy flow of Chi energy throughout the body, was already in use in the area; archaeologists have found stone acupuncture tools dating as far back as 8000 BCE.

The Brahmans of India have sacred texts derived from ancient oral traditions, which detail the use of medicinal plants in Ayurvedic medicine. Archaeologists have traced the ancient herbal knowledge of   Egypt, Persia,   and the Mediterranean back to these Indian, Asian and Chaldean sources, whose knowledge spread throughout the regions through traders and explorers.

Documents dating from 3000 BCE in Egypt discuss healers and the use of herbs in medicine. Sumerian cuneiform tablets dating from 2500-1900 BCE document the use of opium, thyme, saltpeter, pine and licorice to treat medical problems. Syria, Babylon, Persia and Greece all combined their knowledge with the Egyptians in the millennia that followed, and expanded upon its foundations.

In Greece, Theophrastus (372-287 BCE) and Pedanios Discorides (often called the "Father of

Pharmacy, 60 CE) studied over 500 herbs and wrote long treatises on how to properly identify and use herbs for medicinal purposes, giving us The Inquiry Into Plants and Growth of Plants and De Materia Medica, respectively. In Rome, Gaius Plinius Secundus, now known as Pliny the Elder, wrote a 37 volume reference on the known history of herbs. Their knowledge, combined with that of the Ancients, was shared with Europe for hundreds of years and continues to influence much of modern medicine.

With the advent of Christianity in the West, and the ensuing antipathy to all things *pagan*, defined as all things *relating to the country dweller*, knowledge that had been passed down since before the time of Christ was repressed, and the age of new science and reason was embraced. The word villain actually derives from the French word *vilain*, meaning someone who lives in the countryside. The simple beliefs of country-folk, including an oral tradition of tried-an-true herbal healing methods, were literally villainized over a period of centuries.

Nonetheless, it was an exciting time for medicine, and some advances were made while old knowledge was given a new face. In the 5th century CE poems were written in homage to the Willow Tree, its bark made forever bitter after its use in a childhood beating of Jesus Christ. Bitter, and yet infused with the power to heal the pain it once caused. Today, the willow is known by herbalists as a natural source of *salicylic acid*, the active component in modern-day aspirin.

Nicholas Culpepper (1616-1654) is one of the most famous herbalists from recent centuries, having written numerous books during the first half of the 17th Century on herbal medicine. Many of his works were geared to spread knowledge among the general populace, making them both easy to read and distrusted by some of his fellow physicians. His books and remedies are still referenced today by herbalists, much of their efficacy having been proven both by science and time. Culpepper is widely acknowledged for advancing access to herbal knowledge, and despite the errors his work contains it has basically stood the test of time.

Eventually, willow bark was left behind and forgotten as modern man turned away from teas and tinctures to enjoy the ease of the pill form. Herbalism became more of a folk-art, still practiced , while modern science grew adept at synthesizing the chemical constituents from most herbs and herbal formulas into varieties of "new medicines" to treat the growing populations. Meanwhile herbalism continued to grow and flourish.

And yet, today, a vast number of medicines still derive from an original plant form. The World Health Organization reports that at least a quarter of Western medicine derives from plants, and that the modern uses of almost three quarters of those medicines are [the same as] similar to the traditional herbal treatments. Even the most secular medical scientists mourn the loss of the uncharted forests of the world because so many cures for diseases have been found there, and more remain to be found. Ethnobotanists still roam the world to study how cultures use their floral environments hoping to find valuable "keys" – plants that may hold the capacities to cure, or treat, a number of diseases and disorders, especially cancer, diabetes, and heart disease.

Herbalism in the stable outlasted herbalism in the home to a great extent. Until well after the Second World War, many stable managers still used herbal salves and mashes to treat horses in their care. Some of that knowledge has survived, and much of it has been built upon by modern equine herbalists, embracing the infiltration of Eastern medicine into our culture and looking at horse treatment holistically. With the modern sentiment that animals are not beneath man, but interconnected and to be protected, so has the medical treatment progressed to the point where we have animal communicators, massage therapists, and herbalists who are willing to take a closer look at animals as sentient beings with knowledge to share.

Of course there are so many areas throughout our culture and around the world where herbalism has never diminished. Rather it thrives and has been strengthened with the incorporation of Ayurvedic and Chinese Traditional Medicine (TCM) and Native American herbalism. Today this is being much better intertwined with mainstream veterinary practices enhancing the whole field, and especially the outlooks for equestrian health and healing.

Not all herbal wisdom has come to us through human experimentation. Sometimes, the animals themselves have taught us. The Chinese have a folk-tale about the discovery of San Qi, one of their most treasured medicinal herbs, used externally to staunch bleeding and heal wounds.

According to the story, one day a farmer beat a snake to death near his garden. Several days later, he saw the same beaten snake near his hut, and again he beat it until he thought it was dead. When he saw the snake a for a third time a few days later, he beat it again, but this time he watched as the snake slithered amongst some weeds and began to chew on their leaves and stems. The next morning the farmer realized that the weeds were actually a medicinal herb, with the power to heal: the snake was still there, eating the weeds, his wounds already half-healed. German scientists have studied and written extensively about the animal-herbal healing connections in the wild, on land and in the sea, where injured fish, sea otters, and dolphins have been observed rolling amidst sea algae to soothe and heal serious wounds. The Sargasso Sea and other great kelp beds are primary undersea "hospitals" teeming with life and healing potentials.

The ability to self-medicate with herbs is not unique to man. Chimpanzees in the wild have been found to eat medicinal plants when they are ailing – plants which they do not eat on a normal basis. Horses, too, have been observed to seek out the proper herbs in their pasture when the need arises. One of our own horses, 37 years old and suffering from the creaky, aching joints of old age, would often seek out fresh willow in his pasture on his worse days. His younger companion never did – until the day he stepped on a large barn nail from the 1800's in the pasture. For the next week, he stripped the bark off of young willows with uncharacteristic zeal, and submitted happily to morning and evening herbal foot soaks.

In this manner, horses of the past were free to roam on a large acreage and commonly found the herbs and other medicinal plants they needed to stay properly conditioned. Now, though, most horses have restricted access to natural forage, and can not eat the herbs their systems need to stay healthy and combat illness. Pastures have become little more than neatly manicured lawns, and horses cannot access herbs on their own. Herbal formulas address this need. Most herbs are even more palatable and digestible for horses after they have been properly dried, cut and sifted. This means that by making herbal formulas for your horse using dried herbs, you are actually increasing their healing power. This book will teach you how to combine and use herbs most effectively for your horse's benefit.

But first, let's look back briefly at some of the many "old healing formulas" that continue to work for people and animals, and have stood the tests of time. While many folks may use these as "alternative" treatments, in some cases, more people rely on these noted therapeutic treatments as "complementary" to mainstream medicine. These herbal tonics have well-documented histories of providing healing. And what works well for us, often works well for our animals. Many of us use these cleansing formulas as seasonal "tonics" and "preventives" for our horses, as well as ourselves.

"Some researchers believe that the split between herbal and orthodox medicine occurred in 1785. William Withering discovered that, by using precise amounts of the foxglove leaf, he could treat heart failure. He then proceeded to isolate and purify foxglove's active ingredients digitoxin and dioxin. From that point forward, conventional medical and pharmaceutical researchers have believed that the active principle of plants should be extracted, purified, and given in specific dosages to ensure its safety." ~ Enriqueta De Guzman, DVM, MS. *Western Herbal Medicine: Clinical Applications*

CHAPTER TWO

Equine Herbs & Their Properties

"Let your food be your medicine."

Hippocrates, the Father of Medicine, c. 300 BC

Herb gardening and minding meadows filled with herbs are great pleasures, yet not all of us have these advantages. And, even when we do have herb gardens and farms, we cannot always hope to raise all of the herbs we may need for ourselves, our animals, and have enough to make herbal products. We are fortunate to have a range of good herbal suppliers. Many more conventional farmers are setting aside increasing acreage for raising healing herbs. This trend is by no means new, as herbs will survive and thrive where most other things fail. The more we work with herbs the more we appreciate those who harvest, dry, prepare, formulate, and package herbs for our modern needs.

Herbs should always be bought from reputable dealers of food-grade herbs (if you can't find any local suppliers, try Starwest Botanicals, Ameriherb, or Frontier Co-op.) Organic, pesticide free herbs are best whenever possible. When buying dried herbs, for ease of use try herbs that are "cut & sifted". This means that they are clean herbs, which have been cut into small pieces that are easy to handle and mix.

Each herb is a unique, complex chemical factory; indeed, every plant is. All plants contain thousands of chemicals with countless biological activities. It is vital to respect the basic qualities of each plant and study how they complement and interact with each other. These observations gave rise to the earliest formulas. Only recently have we learned that there are many biologically active compounds in herbal medicines.

Herbs play an enormous part in nutritional support, and have been used as part of the healing process since ancient times. We know that herbal nutrients today can add a commanding advantage to healing enabling a horse to regenerate damaged tissue, while empowering the immune system, reducing inflammation, and enhancing metabolic functions, while aiding the overall healing process.

Now which herbs are best for your horses? When and how should they be used? The whole herb produces a useful synergistic effect that can often exceed the benefits of a "magic bullet" of the synthetic counterparts on the market which generally only contain one or two active constituents from an herb. Many horses profit by eating daily supplements of herbs in their feed, while others require special formulas to treat and strengthen the animals against a variety of common ailments and conditions. Older horses particularly enjoy a tasty calorie free handful of herbs sprinkled over their modest grain portions. Herbal wisdom and horse sense join forces here with practical research and natural holistic health care.

"Research and clinical observations reveal that combining modern veterinary medicine with therapeutic nutrition may give better patient response than does either approach alone." ~ Roger V. Kendall, "Therapeutic Nutrition for the Cat, Dog, and Horse." 1998; in *Complementary and Alternative Veterinary Medicine: Principles and Practice.*

Equine Materia Medica

Herbs provide a robust medicine chest for your horses' well-being. Herbs, their diverse fragrances, and essential oils have a profound affect on our wellness and that of our horses. This does not mean that herbs and essential oils replace veterinarian care, but rather can complement it. They simply give the owner and horse more intimate ways of relating and accessing healing on a deeper level. It is best to have veterinary care administered first to deal with what has developed in the physical body safely and with supervision. Once the process begins, then introduce the herbs and essential oils to facilitate healing on the mental and emotional levels so the physical problems are less likely to develop again. As Dr. Allen Schoen notes in the foreword, herbal medicine may need supplement of replace pharmaceuticals if an when strong medicines begin to cause adverse side effects. We have found this particularly true for horsed on strong anti-inflammatories, and many have effectively transitioned to reduced doses because of using our anti-inflammatory herbal formulas.

And remember: **Do not throw herbs at the problem.** Take precious time to evaluate your horses needs, condition, physical, and emotional status. You do not need to give your horse buckets full of herbs to get their benefit. A small synergistic combination of cut and sifted herbs can have an effect within the body in a few doses. If the herbs are powdered you may not need to use more than two tablespoons to help the body heal itself.

Many of these herbs are ones that you could find growing across paddocks or along roadsides, or they might once have been known there. A hundred years ago horses often had free-range of healthy grassed fields. Modern roadsides are not as clean as they once were. Today to get the full benefit of herbs we need to supplement with herbs from clean, pesticide-free lands. Some of these special therapeutic herbs do not grow in every region.

Most of all, plants live in families and have interesting relatives, much like humans and horses. This small equine materia medica we have gathered here reflects plants from around the world useful in horse wellness. Many of these herbs are Asian, Eurasian, and European species that were introduced centuries ago in North America because of their vital therapeutic qualities; some that we might call "weeds," like burdock, cleavers, dandelion, mullein, and nettle, were actually prized herbal medicines to our ancestors, and continue to dazzle us with their healing benefits. Some of these came as seeds aboard the Mayflower carried by hopeful herbalists. Native American herbs like bilberry, boneset, chaparral, echinacea, goldenrod, kelp, and yarrow have been healing people and animals on this continent since earliest times.

Many of our equine herbs are in the composite (or daisy) family, and in the rose and mint families. They are valuable when used alone and even more so in formulation with other herbs developed to target horses myriad needs, and promote ongoing wellness.

The conventional dosages given here are in grams. 5 grams equal approximately 1 teaspoon; 15 grams equal approximately 1 teaspoon; and 230 grams equal approximately 1 cup. Dosage ranges are given for chronic and acute cases. Generally, lower dosages are used by herbalists over long-term periods, for chronic conditions, while higher dosages are used in acute cases to stimulate an immediate response.

Herbal Properties Glossary

Adaptogen: adapts its effect to what the body needs

Alterative: increases overall health & tissue renewal

Analgesic: pain reliever

Anodyne: pain reliever

Antacid: reduces acidity in stomach & gut

Anthelmintic: expels worms & parasites

Antibiotic: kills infections

Antifungal: kills fungal infections

Anti-inflammatory: reduces inflammation in & on the body

Antimicrobial: destroys micro-organisms; i.e. bacteria & fungi

Antiseptic: inhibits growth of bacteria & other infections

Antispasmodic: relieves spasms

Antitussive: relieves coughs

Aperient: gently moves the bowels; gentle laxative

Astringent: draws and binds together soft organic tissues

Aromatic: distinctive fragrant smell

Antiemetic: discourages vomiting

Antioxidant: scavenges free radicals to limit cellular damage

Antirheumatic: relieves arthritis

Antiseptic: cleans wounds and discourages infection by preventing the growth of bacteria

Calmative: sedative & calming

Carminative: helps expel gas to relieve cramps and colic

Demulcent: soothes inflammation

Detoxification: eliminates impurities from the blood & supports the liver

Diaphoretic: increases perspiration

Diuretic: increases and encourages the flow of urine

Electrolytes: natural body salts: sodium bicarbonate, sodium chloride, and potassium chloride

Emetic: causes vomiting

Emmenagogue: promotes menstruation, abortive
Emollient: softens the skin or mucous membranes

Expectorant: expels mucus from the respiratory tract

Febrifuge: reduces fever

Flavonoids: plant constituents that affect healing

Galactagogue: increases the production of milk

Hepatic: drains and cleanses the liver

Immuno-stimulant: stimulates & supports the immune system

Laxative: relieves constipation by promoting bowel movement

Mucilage: demulcent that soothes mucous membranes

Nervine: affects the nervous system

Nutritive: of nutritional or nourishing value

Phytotherapy: therapeutic plant remedies in medicines.

Refrigerant: cools; relieves fever or heat
Sedative: calms and relaxes, soothing nervous tension

Stimulant: energy producing

Stomachic: aids digestion

Styptic: controls bleeding

Tonic: cleanses and promotes healthy bodily functions

Vermifuge: expels worms

Volatile Oils: plant oils easily vaporized with heat or pressure

Vulnerary: heals wounds

"There is something about the outside of a horse that is good for the inside of a man."
~ Winston Churchill

Bilberry

Accinium myrtillus

Parts Used: purple-black, ripe fruit, & green leaves.

This is a small evergreen shrub in the Heath Family, **Ericaceae**

Properties: astringent, antibacterial, antiseptic, laxative, diuretic, refrigerant.

Bilberry has a long tradition as an eye treatment in Europe, even having been used during World War II in Britain to improve airplane pilots' night vision.

Taken internally, bilberry can lower blood pressure behind the eyes, and an herbal remedy for glaucoma and cataracts. This is attributed in large part to the fact that bilberries contain *anthocyanidins* and *proanthocyanidins,* antioxidants that can reduce inflammation, strengthen blood vessels and regulate proper blood flow throughout the body.

Bilberry leaves, like its "cousin" blueberry, are native to North America, and have valuable astringent qualities as a diuretic, and to help prevent bladder or kidney stones, plus they also benefit a variety of digestive conditions. It may be used to help relieve diarrhea and colic, as well as acute liver conditions. Native Americans used blueberry and bilberry leaf teas as an external wash to treat open wounds and sores, and internally to treat urinary tract problems.

Conventional Dosage: 10 to 20 grams per day.

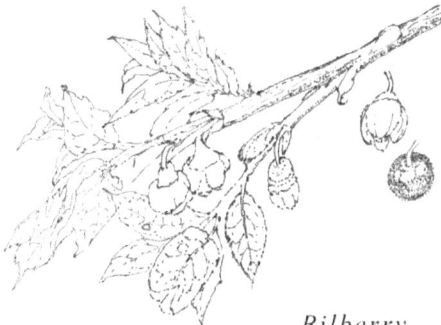

Bilberry

Boneset

Eupatorium perfoliatum,

Parts Used: leaves and new blossoms

This striking perennial herb is in the Composite Family, **Compositae.**

Properties: aperient, antispasmodic, diaphoretic, emetic, febrifuge, stimulant, tonic.

Given to a horse as a dried herb, boneset acts as a tonic and febrifuge, strengthening weakened constitutions and combating recurring fevers.

European research has found that boneset's capacity to stimulate the immune system and combat bacterial infections make boneset a powerful instrument in the herbalist's arsenal. It was used extensively throughout the United States by Native Americans and settlers alike, combating influenza and common colds.

There are varying theories on where boneset's name derived from. It is a fact that it was used to treat "breakbone fever," or dengue. Dengue fever is generally accompanied by joint pain, something which boneset is quite adept at alleviating, along with pains in the bones.

Ancient herbalists used to see an herb's appearance as an indicator of its properties: boneset's very leaves actually appear speared by the stem, much like a modern-day shish ka-bob. Given to horses that have been badly bruised or suffered bone and ligament injuries, boneset may lessen their discomfort.

When taken warm, boneset encourages the passing of fecal matter, and can be used in the manner to help relieve an impacted horse.

Conventional Dosage: 5 to 20 grams per day.

Caution: Boneset should not be taken long-term, as excessive use may lead to liver damage. The dried herb is safer to use than the fresh, as drying reduces some of the potential toxins.

Borage

Borago Officinalis

Parts Used: leaves

This annual herb often self-sows; it is in the Borage Family, **Boraginaceae**

Properties: aperient, diaphoretic, diuretic, demulcent, emollient, febrifuge, galactogogue, refrigerant, stimulant.

Borage is a very soothing mucilaginous herb, both inside and outside the body. It can be used internally to treat fevers and clear respiratory congestion, as well as to soothe and restore stressed adrenal glands. The ancient Romans used it as a mild stimulant, and it has been used throughout the ages as an herbal remedy for depressed spirits.

Externally, borage is extremely useful in reducing bruises and inflamed muscles or joints.

Conventional Dosage: 5 to 10 grams per day.

> **Caution**: Borage over-stimulates the nervous system in large doses; borage should be used with caution, and is not recommended for use with pregnant or nursing mares.

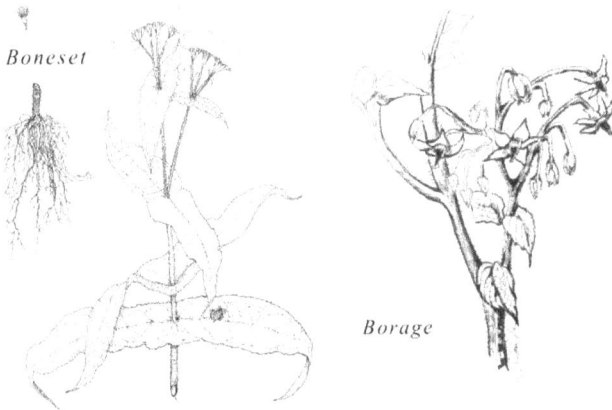

Boneset

Borage

Burdock

Arctium lappa

Parts Used: leaves and roots

This rugged perennial is part of the Composite Family, **Compositae**

Properties: alterative, demulcent, diaphoretic,

diuretic, nutritive.

Burdock is a won-derful blood-cleansing herb that detoxifies the liver, blood, kidneys and entire lymphatic system. Due to these properties, it has a long history of being used to reduce inflammation in joints and muscles, and help lower fevers.

In China, burdock is used to treat arthritis and is one of the foremost detoxifying herbs in both Western and Chinese herbal medicine..

Used externally, burdock root benefits many skin conditions, from rashes and sores, to burns and minor wounds. Infused in oil and applied directly to the skin, burdock also has a reputation for its ability to re-grow and strengthen hair. Leaf poultices relieve skin irritations, sores, and tumors, and have good antiseptic properties.

The Lesser Burdock, *Arctium minus*, can be used in similar ways.

Conventional Dosage: 15 to 30 grams per day.

Burdock is best, as are most herbs, when given in carefully planned and measured formulas that can complement various aspects of the horse's problem(s).

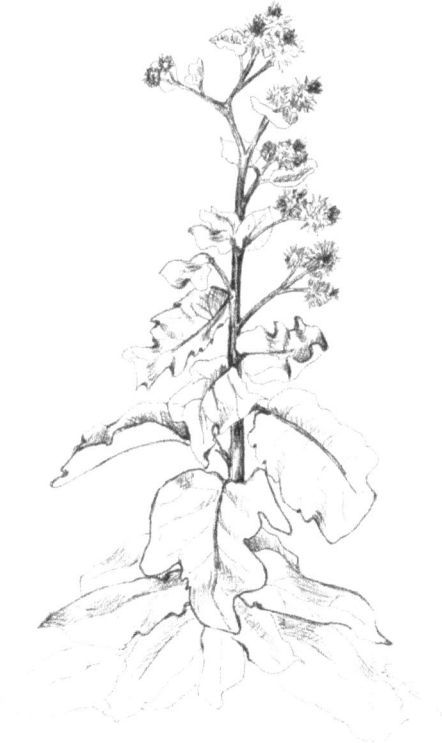

Burdock

Calendula

Calendula officinalis, & C. arvense, a wild species with similar virtues

Parts Used: flower petals
Rugged annual with vivid orange-gold flowers in the Composite Family, **Compositae**

Properties: antispasmodic, anti-inflammatory, antiseptic, detoxifying, mildly estrogenic, astringent, diaphoretic, stimulant, vulnerary.

Calendula, a.k.a. Pot Marigold, is one of the most versatile herbs in Western herbalism; these colorful blossoms, fresh or dried, have vital antiseptic and healing qualities. Calendula stimulates circulation while cleansing the liver and blood, making it very useful in the treatment of bruises and sprains. However, nothing surpasses calendula in its ability to heal and cleanse the skin when used in a wash or taken internally.

Calendula provides effective skin treatments for burns and many rashes, and even proves valuable in treating systemic skin disorders such as eczema, and fungal conditions like ringworm and thrush. Calendula's vibrant, daisy-like flowers certainly encourage cheerfulness and lift the spirits, and are among herbalists favorites!

Conventional Dosage: 20 to 80 grams per day.

Celery

Apium graveolens
Parts Used: seeds, stems, & leaves

This fragrant biennial herb is in the Carrot Family, **Umbelliferae**

Properties: antirheumatic, anti-inflammatory, antispasmodic, carminative, diuretic, emmenagogue, nervine, stimulant, stomachic, tonic.

In Ancient Egypt, celery was used as a tonic to relieve swelling in joints and muscles, to soothe stomachaches and to cure headaches. Celery has a cleansing, tonifying effect on the system that is generally detoxifying. This vegetable, is also a valuable preventive medicine that has been cultivated for more than 3000 years in China and the Middle East.

Today, celery seeds are used primarily to promote regular urination, which in a horse can benefit nerves, arthritis, lung and respiratory ailments, fevers and liver problems. It also helps regulate and lower blood sugar levels and blood pressure. Celery seeds also have a mild sedative, tranquilizing action; the juice, especially when mixed with organic carrot juice, is good to treat chronic illnesses.

Conventional Dosage: 5 to 10 grams per day.

Caution: Not for use with pregnant mares.

Chamomile, German

Matricaria chamomilla, Chamomilla recutita, & Chamemelum nobile, Roman Chamomile, a close relative & used in similar ways
Parts Used: flowers & leaves

Sweet, aromatic daisy self-sows readily & is in the Composite Family, **Compositae**

Properties: anodyne,   anti-inflammatory,

antiallergenic, antispasmodic, carminative, diaphoretic, emmenagogue, nervine, tonic, sedative, stomachic, vulnerary.

Chamomile has long been known for its relaxing, soothing properties. It is used throughout western civilization to calm nerves, promote sleep and help relieve indigestion, colic and headaches. It combines extremely well with other herbs to benefit all illnesses that derive or suffer from stress: general pain and inflammation remedies will benefit from the inclusion of chamomile, which is calming and relaxing to the muscles, nerves and joints in problem areas. Chamomile's aromatic, slightly bitter taste is reminiscent of apples and horses seem to love it!

This versatile herb is a fine insecticide, can relieve eyestrain, and is valuable to treat hay fever and asthma; an external skin application helps relieve eczema and itchy skin patches. Similarly, skin and respiratory allergies can benefit from small doses of chamomile, which will relieve the stress induced by allergies.

Chamomile will also help relieve muscle cramps during menstruation and after foaling, and will increase milk production. As a safe herb to give nursing mares, it can discourage excitability in horses if given while they are young.

"German Chamomile, which contains *spiroether*, a very strong antispasmodic, relaxes tense, aching muscles... relieves irritability and promotes sleep," says London herbalist Andrew Chevallier in *The Encyclopedia of Medicinal Plants.*
Conventional Dosage: 15 to 45 grams per day.

Caution: Not for use with pregnant mares.

Chaparral

Larrea divaricata, Argentinean species & *L. tridentata,* Native American species
Parts Used: leaves, stems

This perennial shrub is in the Caltrop Family, **Zygophyllaceae**

Properties: alterative, antibiotic, antiseptic, antitumor, diuretic, expectorant, laxative, parasiticide, tonic.

Chaparral, a.k.a. Creosote Bush or Greasewood, is a common, thorny shrub, and widely used. Native to North & South America, chaparral grows in the desert, and perhaps because of this, can actually help lower one's body heat and help one stay cool in the desert. It works very well in combination with other herbs to relieve skin rashes and inflammations, including acne, bruises and warts.

Because chaparral contains NDGA, or nordihydroquaiaretic acid, it is a strong respiratory antioxidant, and useful in the treatment of tumors and cancers. Its ability to clear the body of toxins makes it invaluable in circulatory tonics and in the treatment of respiratory ailments. It is especially valuable to relieve arthritis, and to relieve, or even prevent, coughs. Native Americans also used it in anticancer remedies.

Conventional Dosage: 5 to 10 grams per day.

Caution: Use in moderation; not for pregnant or nursing mares.

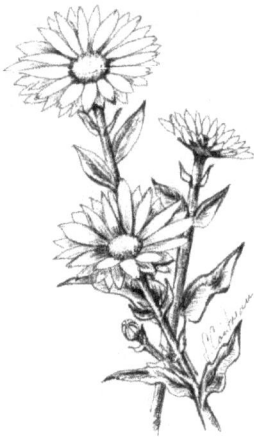

Calendula

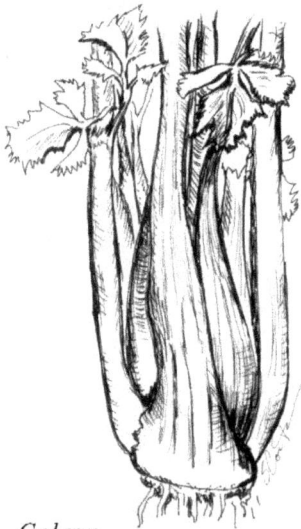

Celery

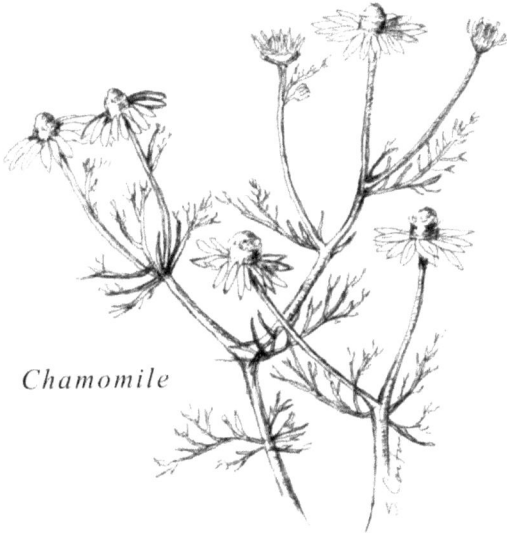

Chamomile

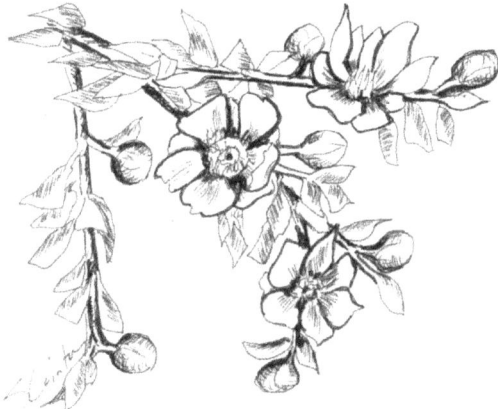

Chapparal

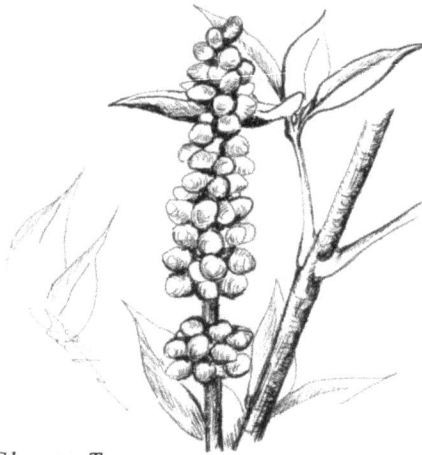

Chaste Tree

Chaste Tree

Agnus castus, Vitex agnus-castus
Parts Used: berry

Properties: adaptogen, emmenagogue, galactogogue, vulnerary.

Deciduous aromatic tree in the Verbena Family, **Verbenaceae**

Among females, chaste tree berries increase the output of progesterone when needed by stimulating the pituitary gland. Conversely, it will lower hormones when they are too high. As an adaptogen, it is reputed to regulate female hormone and menstrual cycles, alleviate many symptoms associated with the menstrual cycle such as irritability, muscle pains, and hormonal mood swings. It is also said to stimulate milk production.

Historically, chaste berry was fed to monks to lessen their sexual urges and interest in the female sex. Presumably, this effect stems from the herb's moderating hormonal properties, and may produce similar effects on a stallion.

Conventional Dosage: 2 to 8 grams per day.

Caution: Not for use with pregnant mares.

Cleavers

Galium aparine
Parts Used: leaves, stems

This common widespread annual is in the Madder Family, **Rubiaceae**

Properties: alterative, aperient, diuretic,

refrigerant, tonic.

Internally, cleavers has shown significant benefits to regulating urination and bowel movements, and cleaning all obstructions and infections from the digestive and eliminative tracts with great efficiency. As such, it is particularly recommended for horses forced to experience extra stall-time, whether due to winter conditions, illness or training restrictions. In any case, cleavers, a.k.a. goose grass or bedstraw, will help the horse resist colic from lack of movement, and keep its bodily functions well in tune.

In recent studies, cleavers has been shown to contain anti-inflammatory and anti-tumor properties, as well as showing a propensity for lowering blood pressure.

Cleavers is taken to detoxify the lymphatic system, especially with cancer treatments; infusions also treat kidney stones, and relieve chronic skin conditions and diseases such as eczema and psoriasis. Cleavers is yet another equine herb that is valuable internally and externally in a variety of therapeutic treatments.

Externally, a salve made from cleavers is

useful in treating dry, itchy skin rashes.

Cleavers close relatives, Lady's Bedstraw, *G. verum*, and Mexican Cleavers, *G orizabense*, are also used in similar applications, as well as to relieve fevers. Mazatecs and other regional Indians also used these herbs to treat intestinal parasites.

Conventional Dosage: 10 to 50 grams per day.

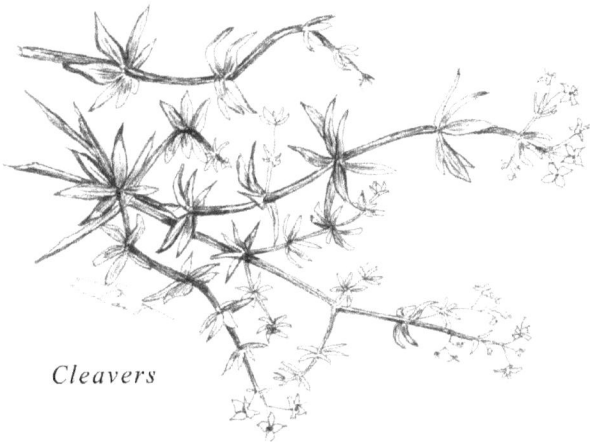

Cleavers

Clover, Red

Trifolium pratense
Parts Used: flowers

This common widespread herb is in the Pea Family, **Leguminosae**

Properties: alterative, anticancer, antispasmodic, antitumor, deobstruant, expectorant, sedative.

Red clover is a mild phytoestrogen, and can be used to treat hormonal imbalances. In small, regular doses, red clover will have a calming effect on a horse, and can even be given to young horses. Red Clover is known to have a contraceptive effect on sheep.

A mild herb, red clover helps relieve inflammation and tones the blood, flushing impurities. Similarly, it is an expectorant and can help soothe lung congestion and coughs. American Indians used Red Clover as a salve to treat burns and other skin irritations, and as a poultice to relieve sore eyes. Indeed, European herbalists used this herb to treat cataracts

Considered a nutritive herb, red clover helps the body assimilate iron and contains a high amount of anti-oxidants, protein and calcium.

Historically among herbalists, clover has long been believed to be valuable in the treatment of cancers and ulcers, perhaps because of its anti-oxidant properties. The National Cancer Institute has more recently confirmed red clover's efficacy as an anti-cancer treatment. To use it as an anti-cancer treatment, red clover may be applied directly to external tumors as a poultice or taken internally as a tea. Red Clover improves the soil, as a nitrogen-fixing legume, and is excellent for grazing and fodder for horses; a sweet source of nectar for honeybees, and is distinguished as Vermont's state flower.

Conventional Dosage: Up to 90 grams per day. Though generally considered a calming herb, excessive doses may have the opposite effect.

Comfrey

Symphytum officinale
Parts Used: leaves only (see Caution below)

A rugged perennial herb in the Borage Family, **Boraginaceae**

Properties: alterative, anti-inflammatory, antitussive, astringent, demulcent, expectorant, tonic, vulnerary.

Comfrey has many valuable applications. The Greek physician Dioscorides wrote about comfrey in his Materia Medica in the 1st century. For hundreds of years, herbalists knew that comfrey helped cells grow and heal, and could be used to good effect in treating wounds, ulcers, broken bones, and torn muscles and tendons. The Latin binomials literally mean "knitting together" and many of this herb's local names refer to its mending qualities, such as bruisewort and knitbone. Comfrey's large leathery leaves lend themselves perfectly to making poultices for soothing countless skin problems from psoriasis and eczema, to bruises and burns, to fungal infections; it will even relieve sprains and stiff aching joints.

Comfrey's efficacy in knitting together ruptures and bones can not be denied. Comfrey contains allantoin, a cell proliferant that is said to clean away necrotic tissue, hastening the growth of new healthy tissue. Allantoin also helps alleviate skin-irritations.

Due to its high mucilage content, comfrey will soothe sore throats and heal a myriad of lung conditions. For the same reason, comfrey is extremely beneficial for the stomach, kidneys and bowels, and works well in tonics to rejuvenate the digestive system. As many equine ailments begin in the stomach, comfrey can be used to good effect in almost any ailment.

Conventional Dosage: 1 to 5 grams per day.

Caution: Not for use with pregnant mares. Comfrey roots contain high amounts of liver-damaging pyrrolizidine alkaloids and should never be used internally; yet when pounded into a gooey mass and applied externally over broken skin as a poultice, they accelerate healing.

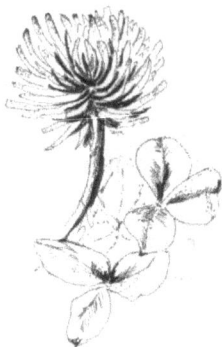

Red Clover

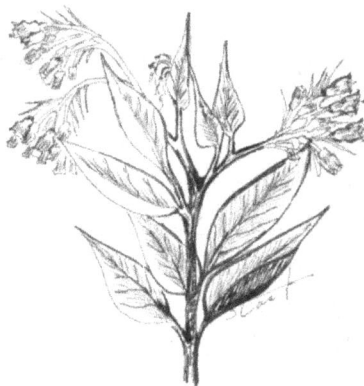

Comfrey

Dandelion
Taraxacum officinale
Parts Used: leaves and root
Ubiquitous perennial herb in the Daisy Family,
Compositae

Properties: alterative, aperient, astringent, cholagogue, detoxifying, diuretic, galactogogue, lithotriptic, stomachic, tonic.

Need someone to blame for your imperfect lawn? Look no further than Greece, the original home of the Dandelion. This wily herb has made its way into lawns and pastures around the globe, perhaps to spread the message that herbalism really isn't any further than your own back yard. Indeed, dandelion is cultivated in France, Germany, and the United States today for the food, beverage, and medicinal virtues increasingly sought by modern commercial needs.

Dandelion's curative properties have been enjoyed since Ancient times; Its Latin name, *Taraxacum officinale*, actually means "official cure of disorders." Dandelion is a powerful detoxifier, and is primarily used to treat problems arising in the digestive system. A potent tonic, dandelion will detoxify the blood and liver as well as cleanse the entire digestive tract. As arthritis and rheumatism in horses often stems from improper digestion, dandelion is a natural remedy for all such ailments.

Because of its strong cleansing properties, dandelion can often help clear skin rashes and allergies, so many of which result from toxins building up in the bloodstream and lymphatic system. For this reason, dandelion is a good herb to add to any formula designed to combat tumors or cysts. It is also reputed to stimulate milk production in nursing mares.

Conventional Dosage: 30 to 90 grams per day.

Devil's Claw

Harpagophytum radix, & H. procumbens
Parts Used: root

Trailing perennial woody African vine in the **Pedaliaceae**

Properties: anodyne, anti-inflammatory, stomachic

Brought to Europe and North America from southern Africa and Madagascar, Devil's Claw has been proven in many studies to reduce inflammation and relieve muscle and joint pain. It is extremely effective when used either internally or externally in the treatment of arthritis and similar chronic conditions, including ligament, tendon, and locomotive disorders. German studies have likened its anti-inflammatory properties to phenylbutazone, with no toxicity or undesirable side-effects. Devil's claw root has also been shown to benefit poor appetites.

Conventional Dosage: 1 to 5 grams per day.

Caution: May stimulate the uterus. Do not use with pregnant mares.

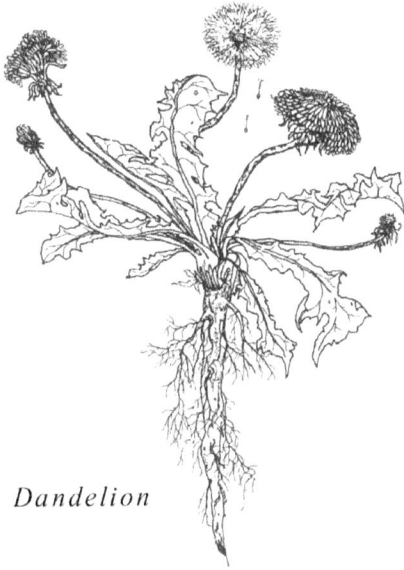

Dandelion

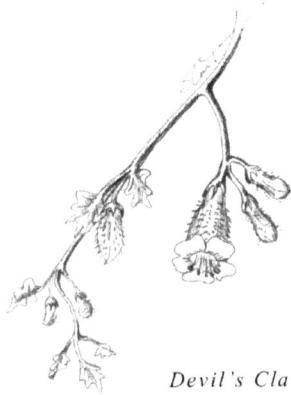

Devil's Claw

Echinacea

Echinacea angustifolia, E. purpurea, & E. pallida
Parts Used: whole herb
Rugged native perennial herb in the Daisy Family,
Compositae
Properties: alterative, antibacterial, antibiotic, antiseptic, antiviral, detoxifying, immune stimulant, vulnerary.

This stunning wildflower is one of the world's most important and well-known medicinal herbs.

An American native, purple coneflower, or echinacea, was used by the Plains Indians as a blood purifier and tonic, as well as to treat toothache and sore throats, and it was eaten as a vegetable. In modern herbal medicine, it is primarily used to combat any kind of bacterial or viral infection. It has been shown to increase white blood cell and T-cell production, and raise the body's overall immune system.

Echinacea works well in conjunction with goldenseal for a full-body cleansing, or with ginseng to stimulate circulation as well.

Studies have shown that echinacea is most effective when taken before any contagion is introduced and in the very first stages of infection.

After two weeks, echinacea's effect on the immune system levels off, and most experts agree that it is best to take echinacea for periods of 2-8 weeks, and then 2-4 week period of "rest" when no echinacea is taken, in order for the herb to continue to work to its full effect.

In cases where a horse has a pronounced fear of crossing streams or walking through water, 2-4 drops of a tincture made of echinacea and skullcap in its water everyday may prove helpful.

Externally, the root was used by Native Americans for centuries as a anti-bacterial poultice to treat festering wounds, insect stings and snake bites.

Conventional Dosage: 10 to 20 grams per day.

Caution: Do not administer to horses with autoimmune disorders or severe allergies.

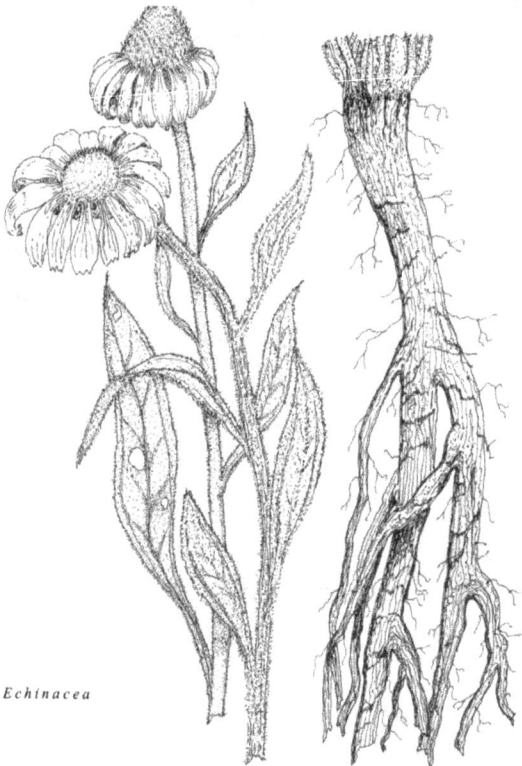

Echinacea

Elecampane

Inula helenium
Parts Used: flower, root

Tall rugged perennial in the Daisy Family,
Compositae

Properties: anti-inflammatory, antiseptic, astringent, carminative, cholagogue, diaphoretic, diuretic, emmenagogue, expectorant, stimulant, tonic

Also known as "Horseheal," elecampane has a long history in veterinary tradition. It infiltrated European tradition from the East, traveling with the horse-traders of Central Asia. Traditional European herbalists used it to help clear out intestinal worms.

In Ancient Egypt, elecampane was used regularly in cooking to aid digestion. Indeed, elecampane stimulates and clears the digestive tract, reducing phlegm production and working as a general energy tonic. Similarly, it will also clear and restore the respiratory and pulmonary systems.

In China and Europe today, elecampane is regularly used by herbalists to clear out mucus and benefit asthma and other chronic lung conditions. Because of its ability to clear the body of mucus and toxins, elecampane can also be used internally to treat many skin conditions to great effect.

It is a warming, restorative, and tonic herb for the lungs most useful for all chesty conditions, and a useful remedy for worms. Its Oriental relative, *Inula japonica,* is known as *Xuan fu hua,* and is used very similarly for diverse treatments.

Conventional Dosage: 5 grams per day.

Caution: Not for use with pregnant mares.

Garlic

Allium sativum
Parts Used: bulb

Ubiquitous bulbous perennial of the Lily Family, **Liliaceae**

Properties: alterative, antibiotic, antiseptic, antispasmodic, carminative, diaphoretic, digestant, diuretic, expectorant, hypotensive, parasiticide, stimulant.

Native to Asia west of the Himalayas, garlic was considered a deity in Ancient Egypt and was a staple of the Egyptian diet used in a myriad of medicinal remedies: for dog and snake bites, bruises, sore throats, toothaches and infected ears. Cloves of garlic have even been found in the tomb of Tutankhamun.

Garlic can be used in equine treatment in any case where the body is in need of detoxification or cleansing. Used throughout the world, garlic is known to ease a plethora of ailments, from a weak metabolism, bad circulation and joint pain, to intestinal worms, respiratory infections and fevers. It has been shown in recent studies to have pronounced anti-cancer and anti-tumor effects. It is also used to regulate both high and low blood pressure, as well as help to lower cholesterol.

Used externally, it is a fine antifungal and antiseptic treatment. This ancient food and medicine is valuable to relieve intestinal parasites, and possesses sufficient antibiotic strength to help treat severe infections.

Conventional Dosage: 15 to 45 grams per day.

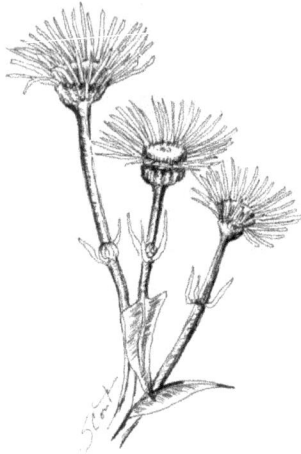

Elecampane

Garlic

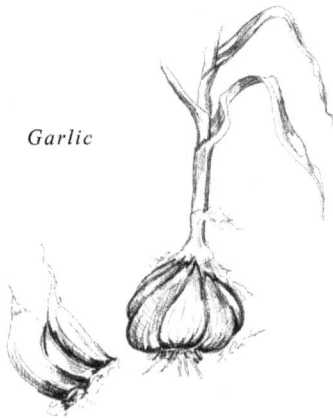

Ginseng, Korean

Panax ginseng

Parts Used: root

Perennial herb in the Ginseng Family, **Araliaceae**

Properties: demulcent, rejuvenative, stimulant, tonic

Known in China as the "Root of Life", Korean Panax Ginseng is unparalleled by other ginsengs in its ability to strengthen and energize the entire body. Ginseng is useful for strengthening the immune system, in the treatment of Lyme Disease, arthritis, and any otherwise weakened condition. Lethargic, malnourished, depressed and abused horses are all generally good candidates for remedies containing ginseng. As they age, horses will have a better chance at longevity with a bit of ginseng added to their regular diet.

Ginseng is also currently under scientific examination as an anti-cancer remedy. Written around 100 B.C. in China, *The Herbal Classic of the Divine Ploughman* mentions ginseng's ability to fortify the body and fight cancer. Modern western science is finally catching up with Eastern medicine, and studies are finding that ginseng derivatives do in fact improve the survival and recovery rates chances of animals stricken with cancer.

This herb is extensively cultivated, along with the other species, and is one of the most popular in Chinese, Japanese, Korean, and Russian traditional medicines. This specie is Ren Shen in TCM, while the American ginseng, *Panax quinquefolium*, is Xi Yang Shen, and is prized to tonify the lungs. It is also cultivated in China for extensive medicinal needs.

Conventional Dosage: 5 to 20 grams per day.

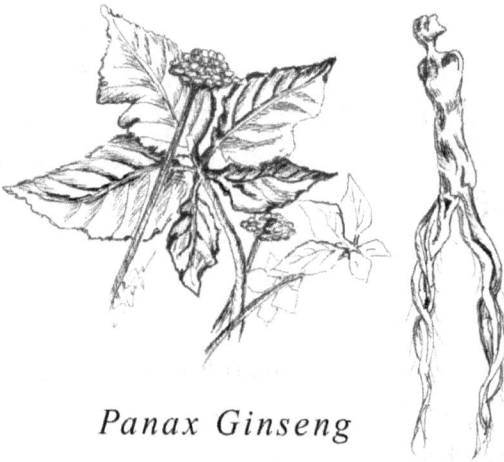

Panax Ginseng

Goldenrod

Solidago Canadensis, odoratum, & species
Rugged perennial herbs in the Daisy Family,
Compositae

Parts Used: leaves

Properties: antioxidant, astringent, carminative,
diaphoretic, diuretic, stimulant

Horses love the flavor of anise-like goldenrod,
and it can be used to enhance an herbal mixture's
appeal. Perhaps in part because of its sweet
nature, goldenrod works well to strengthen the
stomach and help prevent colic and flatulence.
Often wrongly accused of causing seasonal pollen
allergies, goldenrod can in fact help alleviate
them, significantly reducing runny noses.
Goldenrod's *saponins* act specifically against
yeast and fungal infections, even common
problems like cystitis, and can help break up and
relieve bladder and kidney stones. Goldenrod
makes a stimulating tea by steeping a handful of
dried, or two handfuls of fresh herbs in three
cups of boiling water for ten minutes. This is a
good aid to digestion and can be cooled and
added to the horse's water or sprinkled over its
grains. Or, add a small handful of dried goldenrod

to the horse's dry feed when necessary.

In traditional European medicine, goldenrod is recognized as "a sovereign wound-herb, inferior to none, both for inward and outward use," according to Culpepper. It can be used externally to wash and heal wounds and burns, and internally as a diuretic to cleanse the kidneys and urinary tract.

Conventional Dosage: 10 to 20 grams per day.

Hawthorn

Crataegus oxyacantha & *C. monogyna*
Showy deciduous shrub or small tree in the Rose Family, **Rosaceae**

Parts Used: berries, flowers, leaves

Properties: astringent, antidiarrhetic, antispasmodic, digestant, sedative, tonic.

Hawthorn is a well-reputed remedy for all things relating to the heart and circulatory system, and has been used by Native Americans in this capacity, as well as to treat arthritis and muscle soreness. It strengthens and helps heal damaged collagen in the tendons and ligaments, offsetting the damaging effects of arthritic inflammation. In modern herbalism, it is used to treat heart murmurs and irregularities, both low and high blood pressure, pulmonary inflammation and heart disease, strengthening the heartbeat. The Chinese have long used hawthorn berries to alleviate poor digestion derived from circulatory troubles: used regularly in small doses, Hawthorn will gently improve circulation throughout the entire body.

Hawthorn, correspondingly, strengthens the equine cardiac system, as this is one of the best tonics and stimulants for the circulatory system, heart, and blood pressure. A small handful of dried leaves, buds, and berries added to a horse's diet is a good therapeutic ammendment, if needed.

Conventional Dosage: 5 to 10 grams per day.

Horsetail

Equisetum arvense
Parts Used: leaves, stems

This fern ally is a rugged perennial in the Horsetail Family, **Equisetaceae**

Properties: antibiotic, astringent, diuretic, styptic

This slender plant resembling asparagus, horsetail is a member of the ancient family of immense flora that dominated the earth some 400 million years ago. Lucky for us, it is fairly common, and has chosen to stick around, sharing its invaluable medicinal qualities. In South America, the tallest of these 30 unique species *E. giganteum,* can grow to a height of 30 feet. Also known as "bottlebrush" and "scouring rush" because the Native Americans used the stems to scrub utensils and dishes, horsetail contains large amounts of silica and is extremely beneficial to horses in cases of skin allergies and suppressed urination.

Because of this and its high content of silicon, horsetail can also be used in any treatment that is designed to develop healthy hooves, bones or joints. Horsetail is effectively used in poultices, teas and decoctions (added to the horse's water,) and chopped fine fresh or dried over regular feed, as needed. A decoction of horsetail added to the horse's bath can benefit slow-healing sprains and fractures, and relieve some skin conditions, especially eczema. Native Americans used horsetail rush to treat their horses' chronic swelling of the legs, rheumatic and arthritic problems, and to help speed repair of damaged connective tissue, improving natural elasticity.

Horsetail contains aconitic acid and can be used in both teas and washes to stop internal or external bleeding, thus a fine styptic, as well as to help rebuild damaged kidneys and livers.

Conventional Dosage: 5 to 15 grams per day.

Caution: Do not use horsetail for more than 6 weeks except under care and with the proper herbal complements, as this herb may cause irritation in the digestive tract.

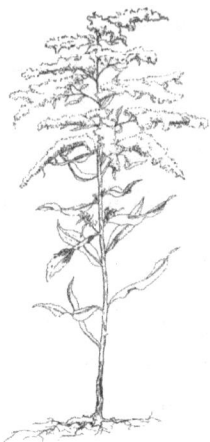
Goldenrod

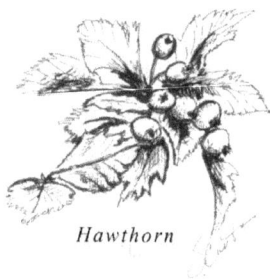
Hawthorn

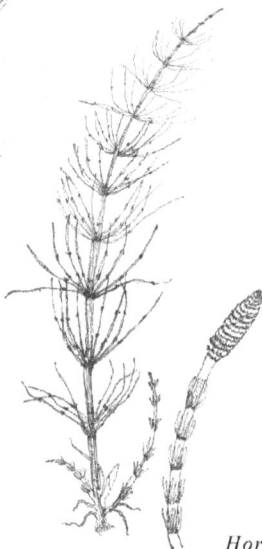
Horsetail

Kelp

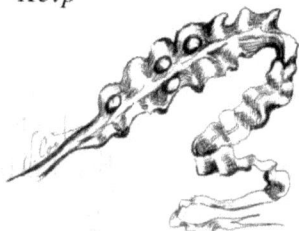

Kelp

Bladderwrack, *Fucus vesiculosis,* & Kelp, *Laminaria digitata,* & *L. saccharina*
Parts Used: all

Rugged perennial seaweed (algae) of the Kelp Family, **Laminariaceae**

Properties: demulcent, emollient, diuretic, nutritive, tonic.

These ancient sea algae are common in Pacific and Atlantic coastal waters. They have long been used by Native Americans as foods and soothing medicines, especially to treat rheumatism, sore ligaments and muscles, and to bathe their horses in kelp decoctions. Both kelps and bladderwracks were used as winter feed for Native Americans' horses and cattle, and to treat a host of problems for human and beast.

Kelp is a fabulous source of iodine, alkali, calcium and silicon, all of which are very good for horses. Use as a general digestive aid and nutritional supplement, and to improve blood and hoof quality. In the winter, a bit of kelp in your horse's feed may encourage hydration and act as a deterrent against colic. Contemporary scientific evidence shows that these sea algae contain *polysaccharides* and minerals (especially iodine) that are immune stimulants. Also *aligns* derived from kelp are soothing to the mucous membranes, especially the respiratory tract, and *emollients,* which soften the skin.

Conventional Dosage: 10 to 200 grams per day.

Caution: Not advised during pregnancy. Use sparingly while nursing foal.

Marshmallow

Althea Officinalis
Parts Used: root, leaves; whole plant

Rugged perennial of marshy regions in the Mallow Family, **Malvaceae**

Properties: alterative, anti-inflammatory, demulcent, diuretic, emollient, expectorant, galactogogue, laxative, lithotriptic, tonic, vulnerary.

The emperor Charlemagne (742-814 A.D.) appreciated marshmallow and ordered it to be cultivated. The Greek word *Althea* means, "to heal" and the herb has provided countless medicines since ancient times. Native to Europe and Asia, marshmallow was introduced to the Ancient Egyptians from Syria, where it was used to treat gastric disorders. Extremely easy to digest, marshmallow has the ability to soothe and rehabilitate the kidney, colon and urinary tract with its lubricating properties. Similarly, it may be used to alleviate colic and diarrhea.

Marshmallow also has anti-inflammatory properties, and is extremely useful in the treatment of muscle and joint problems, as well as against any lung irritations or coughs. Culpepper praises the roots for "hurts, bruises, falls, blows, sprains, or disjointed limbs, or any swelling pain, or ache in the muscles, sinews or arteries." Externally, a strong marshmallow tea makes a soothing, softening wash for burns and scabs, while taking away the healing itch.

A very safe, gentle herb, it is highly recommended for stimulating the production of milk in nursing mares. Use a small handful, perhaps 6-ounces, of dried diced root daily in the horse feed.

Conventional Dosage: 15 to 75 grams per day.

Caution: Do not give to a pregnant horse until after foaling - hastens birth!

Meadowsweet

Filipendula (Spiroea) ulmaria
Parts Used: leaves & flowering tops

Tall rugged perennial in the Rose Family, **Rosaceae**

Properties: anodyne, febrifuge, anti-inflammatory, antirheumatic, antiseptic, diurectic

Known as "meadwort" during the Middle Ages, then Queen of the Meadow, this tall graceful herb was sacred to the Druids, and a choice "strewing herb" inside residences. Meadowsweet was esteemed by herbalists throughout the ages for its pain-relieving qualities and abilities to reduce fevers and remedy flu symptoms. Its high tannin content and astringent qualities make is effective in treating diarrhea and some urinary tract infections. Many herbalists recommend it to relieve heartburn and gastritis. Its major benefit may be to relieve acidity.

Meadowsweet contains *salicylic acid*, first identified and obtained in 1835, and as such is useful in the same cases one would employ aspirin: for fevers, aches and pains. Culpepper recommended it in large quantities to help heal wounds and promote the breaking of fevers. Horses respond well to its gentle properties, and it combines well with white willow and chamomile as a remedy to chronic arthritis.

Use a large handful, perhaps 8- to 9-ounces, of fried herb in the horse feed as needed; or 2-handfuls of fresh-cut herb mixed into the horse feed. Fresh or dried herbs can also be steeped in a pint of boiling water; cooled; then added to the horse water or feed.

Conventional Dosage: 10 to 30 grams per day.

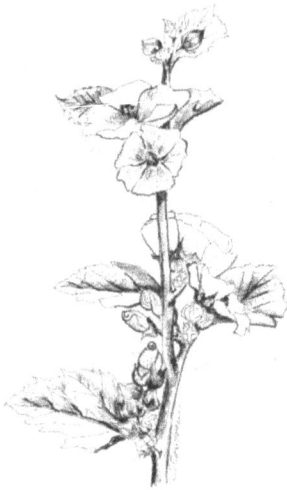
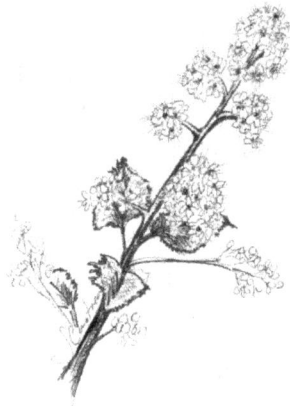

Marshmallow   *Meadowsweet*

Milk Thistle

Silybum marianum
Parts Used: seeds

Tall spiny biennial in the Daisy Family, **Compositae**

Properties: antidepressant, demulcent, galactagogue, hepatoprotective, tonic.

Milk thistle seeds, another Eurasian herb, contain *hesperidin* and *silymarin*, cell-strengthening antioxidants, and are the most powerful herb one can use to cleanse and treat liver. Milk thistle has been proven in clinical studies to significantly regenerate liver tissue. A potent preventative and corrective treatment for liver damage of any kind, milk thistle is, nonetheless, a safe herb for extended use. Just a couple of seeds a day will help protect the liver from toxins and help counteract the liver damage a horse may experience when on the stronger anti-inflammatory medications.

Milk thistle seeds are an excellent spring tonic and should be given for a month to 6 weeks, as the body absorbs their essence slowly. Grind the seeds well before adding them to the feed. This is especially good for horses and ponies that might be suffering from liver damage due to prolonged use of drugs, or from worming difficulties. Milk thistle can also improve appetite and help prevent colic, and was used for centuries in Europe by wet-nurses to improve their milk production.

Conventional Dosage: 5 to 45 grams per day (add to evening feed)

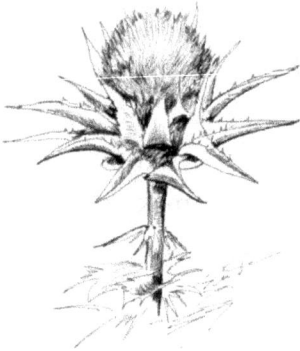

Milk Thistle

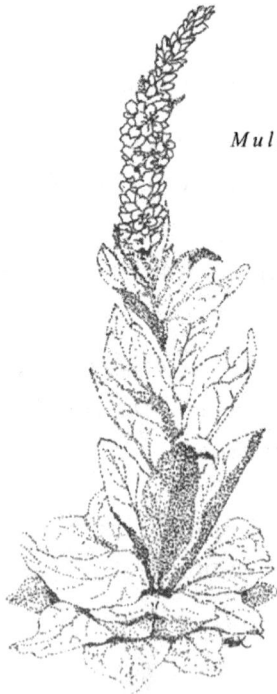

Mullein

Mullein

Verbascum blattaria, V. thapsus
Parts Used: leaves & flowers

Tall hairy(velvety) biennial in the Snapdragon Family, **Scrophulariaceae**

Properties: anodyne, astringent, antispasmodic, demulcent, diuretic, emollient, expectorant, pectoral, vulnerary.

Mullein leaves were used by Native Americans, who quickly adapted this Eurasian herb, to alleviate a variety of lung ailments, from whooping cough and bronchitis, to pneumonia, asthma, and influenza; leaves were applied externally as wound dressings. Large woolly leaves were excellent to line shoes and moccasins. Early colonists taught the Indians the therapeutic virtues of smoking dried mullein leaves to treat respiratory ailments. Mullein has a very mild sedative effect; this combined with its ability to expel mucus and remedy coughs makes it an invaluable treatment for seasonal allergies and chronic coughs. For a well-rounded respiratory treatment, combine mullein with stinging nettle.

Mullein is also reputed to expel tapeworms, though the authors have not tried this usage. Large concentrations of natural mucilage in this herb makes it a soothing expectorant. The yellow flowers in olive oil are a noted pain-relief remedy for earache Externally, a warm poultice or salve made from mullein steeped in apple-cider vinegar will help bruises, pains and aches fade away.

Conventional Dosage: 30 to 90 grams per day.

Nettle, Stinging

Urtica dioica
Parts Used: leaves & aerial parts

Tall hairy perennial herb in the Nettle Family, **Urticaceae**

Properties: anti-inflammatory, astringent, diuretic, expectorant, galactagogue, hemostatic, nutritive, pectoral, tonic.

Nettle is one of the highest sources of iron and easily used by the body; it helps restore the shine and dappling in a horse's coat. The burning, stinging qualities received from the urtic acid when handling the fresh plant act as a counterirritant, causing increased blood flow to the area, and thereby reducing inflammation. Nettles are also a fine tonic and some horses may become more frisky and lively with this herb added to their diet.

Like mullein, another Eurasian herb in origin, stinging nettle is quite useful in most respiratory ailments, expelling mucus and easing congestion in both the lungs and sinuses. It is an effective antihistamine, its own gentle histamines attaching to the body's receptor sites and preventing stronger allergic reactions. As a diuretic and tonic, it will cleanse and calm the kidneys and urinary system while raising a horse's energy. Stinging nettle leaf may also be a new therapeutic option for prolonging remission in inflammatory bowel disease, according to current research.

Rich in iron and potassium, stinging nettle is well-known throughout Europe for its ability to purify and tone blood and the circulatory system. Furthermore, its energizing and anti-inflammatory properties also make stinging nettle a valuable ingredient in any joint or arthritis therapy, and it has long been used both internally as a tea and externally as a poultice by Native

Americans in this capacity.

To improve the quality of your horse's hair and to soothe sore muscles, make a strong infusion of stinging nettles and use it as a rinse at the end of your horse's bath, or after a hard ride.

Stinging nettles, along with red raspberry, are an ideal supplement to a pregnant mare's diet, providing many of the vital nutrients she needs. In particular, nettles are very high in vitamin K, which is very important for a foal's proper growth and development. Dosage may vary from a generous pile of cut, wilted nettles greens given daily, to a handful or 5- to 6-ounces of dried herb added to the regular feed daily.

Conventional Dosage: 15 to 150 grams per day.

Caution: Some horses may break out in a slight "nettle rash" of raised bumps just under the skin; this normally disappears within 8 to 24-hours without problem. If your horse is sensitive, discontinue use of nettles.

Peppermint

Mentha piperita
Parts Used: leaves and aerial plant parts
Highly aromatic perennial herb in the Mint Family,
Labiatae

Properties: alterative, aromatic, calmative, carminative, diaphoretic, stomachic.

The mint family gives us more than 25 distinctive species and hundreds of unique varieties and hybrids to work with; many share similar characteristics and chemical properties. Peppermint and spearmint, *M. spicata,* are the best known in America, where farmers cultivate almost 100,000 acres annually.

Peppermint was cultivated in Egyptian gardens in ancient times, and continues to be drunk as a tea in the Middle East for its digestive and cooling properties. Indeed, it has been used in the Middle East as a healing herb for over 3000 years, and was one of the favored herbs of physician Abu Mansur Mowafik, who wrote a treatise on pharmacology 1600 years before the birth of Christ. These same properties make it a natural remedy for colds, fevers, and flus. Grandmothers throughout the world know that a bit of peppermint in a cup of tea or a bowl of rice is guaranteed to bring some relief to a little one's upset tummy or fever, soothing cramps and nausea. This is an herb that is well-loved by horses when dried, and can be added daily to a horse's feed to support proper digestion and help prevent colic.

Native American aromatic mints like bee balm, *Monarda didyma,* wild bergamot, *M. fistulosa,* horsemint, *M. punctata,* and horse balm, *Collinsonia canadensis,* are used very similarly in these treatments, and have a long history of therapeutic use for Indian ponies and horses. Dosage: 1 or 2-handfuls of fresh leaves daily, or a small handful of dried leaves and blossoms daily added to the horse feed.

Conventional Dosage: 15 to 150 grams per day.

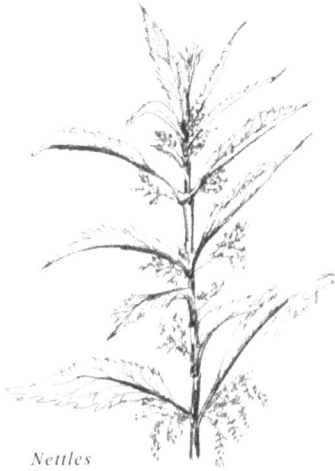

Nettles

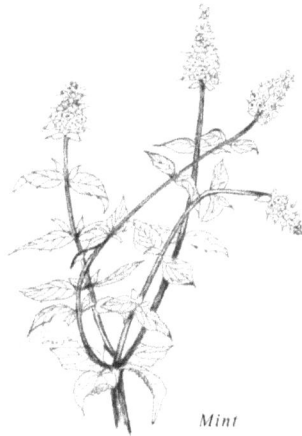

Mint

Plantain

Plantago major, English Planatain, *P lanceolata,* &
Hoary Plantain, *P. media*
Parts Used: leaves and seeds
Ubiquitous perennials in their own Plantain
Family, **Plantaginaceae**

Properties: alterative, anti-inflammatory, antiseptic, astringent, diuretic, emollient, expectorant, refrigerant, vulnerary.

Plantain is another Eurasian introduced herb brought by the early settlers in the 1600s because of its many uses. The eastern Indians called it "white man's foot" because it so quickly spread everywhere the settlers went, and most native tribal herbalists were quick to apply its many therapeutic benefits. Perhaps its most important use is that when crushed into a poultice it has the fantastic ability to heal all manner of skin injuries. It can draw out the poisons from insect and spider bites, and quickly relieves burns, cuts and wounds. As an antiseptic, its anti-microbial properties will keep a wound clean, in addition to cooling the skin and soothing the pain.

Taken internally, plantain's diuretic properties make it useful in treating all types of kidney, urinary and digestive tract infections, as well as colic. Traditionally, it has also been used to treat cancer. *Che qian cao, P. asiatica,* is used in Chinese medicine as a gentle diuretic and to relieve mucus conditions. Several species of native American plantains are extensively used in American Indian herbal skin and respiratory treatments, and to relieve pain and fatigue.

Dosage: a small handful of dried leaves, or two handful of fresh leaves, daily with horse feed.

Conventional Dosage: 15 to 75 grams per day.

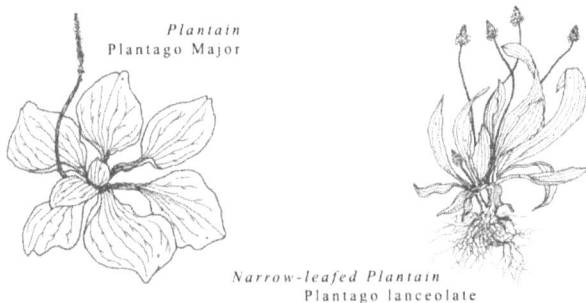

Plantain
Plantago Major

Narrow-leafed Plantain
Plantago lanceolate

Raspberry

Rubus idaeus
Parts Used: leaves

Bristly perennial shrubs in the Rose Family, **Rosaceae**

Properties: alterative, antispasmodic, astringent, hemostatic, parturient, stimulant, tonic.

Raspberry leaves are one of the few herbs that are not only safe for a pregnant mare to eat, but highly recommended in small, regular doses by many herbalists as it can help prevent miscarriage. Raspberry is reputed to ease childbearing by strengthening the uterine muscles. Indeed, it is also beneficial during the menstrual cycle, easing cramps and calming the vaginal muscles.

As a hemostatic, is will prevent excessive bleeding in many situations, and can also be used to calm diarrhea. In Russian folk medicine, a decoction of the leaves is used as a cold and congestion remedy. Numerous Native American species of raspberries and their close relatives were used regionally by native people for foods and the therapeutic leaves and root bark served to treat everything from sore eyes and topical wounds, to easing childbirth and treating cancerous tumors.

Conventional Dosage: 15 to 100 grams per day will help relieve mouth problems, strengthen female reproductive organs and calm digestive troubles. Small doses of raspberry leaves are sometimes given during the last three weeks of pregnancy to strengthen the uterus and ease the birthing.

Thyme

Thymus vulgaris & species
Parts Used: leaves, stems, & blossoms

Aromatic creeping perennial herb in the Mint Family, **Labiatae**

Properties: antiseptic, antispasmodic, carminative, emmenagogue, stimulant, tonic.

Thyme was a symbol of courage in medieval times, and this herbal tea was believed to protect the dreamer from nightmares and daymares. Today's mare benefits from its antiseptic qualities to cleanse the uterine system after birthing. The Ancient Greeks honored thyme as a sacred herb, burning it for incense as a temple sacrifice. Traditionally, thyme was used in all manner of headaches, emotional disorders, and sinus troubles. Culpepper recommended it to purge "the body of phlegm, and it is an excellent remedy for shortness of breath." In the treatment of horses, it is a particularly valuable anti-inflammatory for muscle and joint pains, and a general remedy for rheumatism. As it aids digestion and eases a variety of aches and pains, thyme can benefit almost any chronic equine ailment.

Many species of thyme, each with different volatile oil contents, tannins, and flavonoids are used therapeutically to tonify internal organs and support the immune system. Thyme is a fine antiseptic tonic to treat respiratory problems, and externally to treat spider and insect bites, thrush and other common fungal infections. Infusions of thyme are excellent to bathe the horse.

Thyme was used throughout Europe in households as a favorite strewing herb, along with rosemary, sage and lavender. Scattered on the floor and walked upon, thyme's antiseptic properties discouraged disease while permeating the house with its gentle, pine-like fragrance; this is further enhanced by its insecticidal properties. Try sprinkling a bit among your horse's bedding to bring in a bit of the outdoors and relax your horse.

Conventional Dosage: 5 to 20 grams per day.

Caution: Being an emmenagogue, thyme is not recommended for use with pregnant mares.

White Willow

Salix Alba
Parts Used: bark & leaves

Tall, rugged tree in the Willow Family, **Salicaceae**

Properties: anodyne, anti-inflammatory, astringent, febrifuge, tonic.

Over 300 species of willow grow around the northern temperate and arctic zones where their bark and leaves have served people and animals reservoirs of healing and pain relief. The Greek physician Dioscorides wrote in the first century A.D. about willow's ability to reduce fevers, headaches, and pains.

Willow bark contains the glucoside *salicin*, that becomes *salicylic acid*, and is the one of the original sources of aspirin, *acetylsalicylic acid*. Modern aspirin was developed from willow and meadowsweet. In its herbal form, willow is a gentler, but more effective equine therapy. As with aspirin, willow bark will reduce fevers, joint and muscle inflammation, and benefit the heart.

In European tradition, willow bark was used to treat gas and colic, as well as suppressed urine. Externally, willow may be added to braces or washes to hydrate and clean wounds, sores and burns. Native Americans used willow twigs as chew sticks and dentifrices to relieve toothache, and treat mouth and gum problems. This was also a fine source of vitamin C and other trace minerals. Native herbalists pounded willow bark into soothing poultices as wound dressings and to relieve joint pains for people, dogs, and horses alike. Native children knew the willows as the "headache trees" and the "toothbrush trees" favoring wet regions.

Conventional Dosage: 10 to 50 grams per day or 2 handfuls of fresh leaves daily added to the horse feed; a decoction of willow bark is excellent to massage sore muscles and ease away cramps.

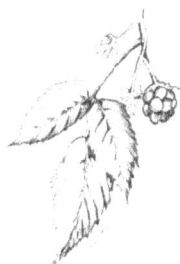

Raspberry

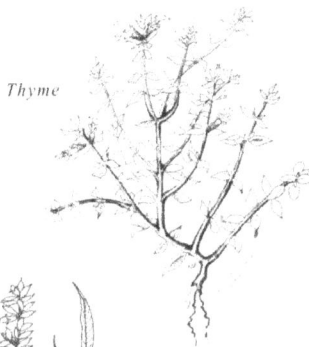

Thyme

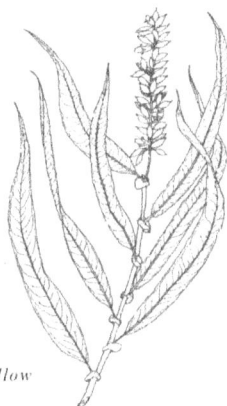

Willow

Yarrow

Achillea millefollium
Parts Used: flowers, leaves

Rugged, feathery perennial in the Composite (Daisy) Family, **Compositae**

Properties: alterative, antibacterial, antispasmodic, astringent, carminative, diaphoretic, diuretic, hemostatic, tonic.

Yarrow has been used throughout the world for thousands of years. It is a fantastic all-around herb, with cleansing and healing properties for the entire body, and is useful both internally and externally. Native Americans used yarrow to relieve chronic fatigue and weakness, as a wound dressing, and to stimulate circulation.

Yarrow was among the first herbs brought to America by our early ancestors, who had no way of knowing it already existed here. Yarrow is an ancient herb found worldwide and employed in divination and medicinal treatments by perhaps every culture on the globe.

Internally, yarrow will cleanse the blood and strengthen many body organs, including the lungs. It helps purge toxins from the blood and kidneys, as well as bacteria and viruses from the body, making it extremely useful in the treatment of any cold or flu, and most childhood illnesses. It stops excessive bleeding, inside and out: use it to lessen excessive menstruation, heal internal injuries, and relieve bruises.

Externally, yarrow's ability to speed the clotting process makes it an ideal herb to heal all sorts of cuts and wounds. Simply make a tea or poultice of the dried herb or use fresh, slightly crushed, leaves and place directly on the wound to stem bleeding.

Conventional Dosage: 5 to 50 grams per day.

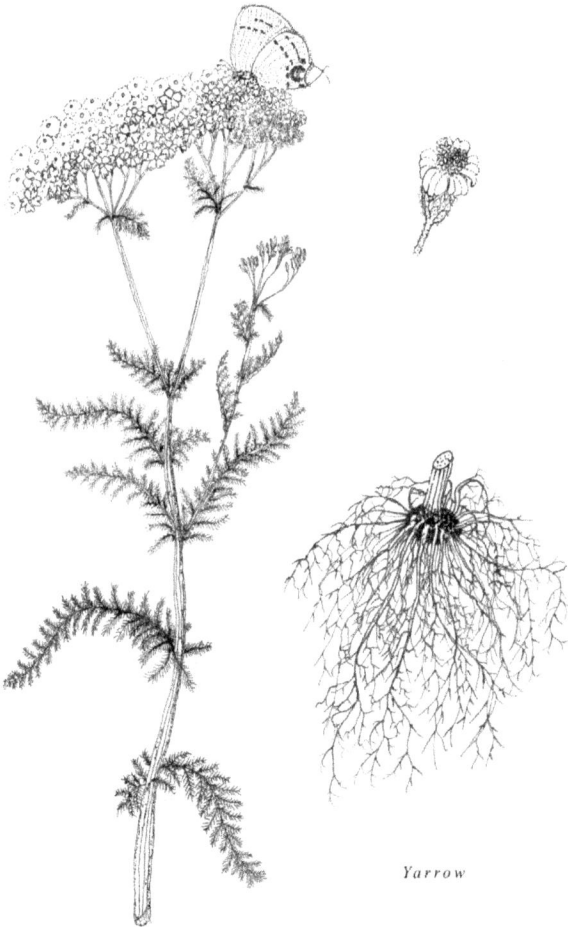

Yarrow

CHAPTER THREE

Oils in Medicine & Aromatherapy

"...and God took a handful of Southerly wind, blew his breath over it, and created the horse." ~
Bedouin Legend

Essential oils have been used since before the time of Christ to heal and protect people from illness. The Ancient Egyptians used essential oils, resins and gums to preserve the dead over 5000 years ago. The Greeks learned from the Egyptians, using essential oils like Myrhh to help mend wound and sooth injuries at the Olympics. During the great plagues of Europe, perfumers were villainized by the church and the public, as they rarely caught the dreaded illness – the church cast them in league with Satan, when in fact they were merely protected by the anti-bacterial and antiseptic properties of oils like

Lavender, Benzoin and Myrhh.

The modern practice of aromatherapy as we know it refers both to the inhalation and direct application of essential oils. A French chemist specializing in the creation of perfumes named René-Maurice Gattefossé was the first person to use the term "aromatherapy." In a lab accident, he became intimately acquainted with the healing powers of lavender: burned in a fragrance lab explosion, he submerged his arm in lavender oil to dull the heat. He noticed that it also subdued the pain, and his arm seemed to heal faster than ever before. This spurred him on to further investigate the medicinal properties of essential oils, and in 1928 he published a book of his findings titled "*Aromatherapie.*"

His work remained largely unknown, though it inspired a few adventurous doctors to experiment with his findings. In 1964, a French surgeon named Dr. Jean Valnet published a book on essential oils by the same name as Gattefossé, covering his own experiments using oils to treat patients with emotional problems and physically-wounded soldiers during the second World War. The world was finally ready for "*Aromatherapie*" and the field has continued to grow and gain momentum as a valid medicinal treatment since its publication, with new research every year showing that essential oils have true medicinal value.

As their name implies, most essential oil properties closely mirror those of their parent plants, in extreme concentrated form. It takes around four million jasmine flowers to create one pound of essential oil. Molecularly, essential oils are quite tiny, smaller than carrier oils, which allows them to absorb directly into the blood stream. Lavender, the herb recommended for sleep pillows and nighttime baby baths, yields an essential oil that is calming both for the mind and the body: lavender essential oil can speed healing and lessen pain. Horses are generally soothed by lavender, and we often put lavender on our wrists before riding. Many oils, including Lavender, also have antiseptic properties which stem from their role in the living plant, where they help deter bacterial and fungal invasions.

Essential oils work on several levels. When essential oils are inhaled, they work the sensual, olfactory level, stimulating the olfactory receptor cells and transmitting the cellular information of the oil properties to the limbic system, the emotional powerhouse of the brain, which is connected to the endocrine system of the body, as well as the respiratory and circulatory systems. From there, the information is transmitted to the entire body.

Carrier Oils

Many essential oils are too potent to be used full strength on the skin. Carrier oils allow essential oils to be applied directly to the skin. By diluting essential oils, which have extremely small molecules, with carrier oils, which have larger, fatty cells, essential oils may be used on the body. When applied directly to the body in a carrier oil, the smaller molecules of the essential oils are absorbed through the skin and reach the bloodstream within hours, or sometimes minutes depending on the oil being used. The carrier oil remains in the outer layers of the skin, acting as a moisturizer.

It is very important to match your carrier oil to your specific needs. Carrier oils have different shelf lifes, thicknesses, odors, and even herbal properties. There are many oils on the market these days -- from the more common canola, soy, and sunflower to the lesser known walnut, Grapeseed and more. In a pinch most oils will do, but there are six oils that are perhaps used the most in aromatherapy and massage work. These are: almond oil, apricot oil, avocado oil, grapeseed oil, jojoba oil and olive oil.

Almond and **apricot** are both relatively light oils, and absorb nicely when massaged into the skin. Their shelf life is the shortest of the six. A small amount of vitamin E added to your blend will extend the life of these oils without thickening them.

Avocado is quite rich and thick, and is fantastic for very dry skin, as is **olive** oil. Olive oil is an old favorite among herbalists due to its long shelf life and healing, nutritive properties. It does have a stronger smell, but this is often overcome when herbs are infused in it. Olive oil can be stored for 12-18 months at room temperature.

Jojoba oil is probably the best oil for the skin and hair. It is a solid oil at room temperature, and as such has an extremely long shelf life. Add it to your blends to increase shelf life and condition hair & skin. **Grapeseed** oil is a light oil with anti-inflammatory properties, making it the ideal carrier oil for liniments and wound salves.

Modern Extraction Methods

Choosing between different manufacturers of essential oils, and their different extraction methods, can be confusing. Make sure that all your essential oils are aromatherapy grade, and not just for fragrance use only. Aura Cacia and Aromavera are both very good suppliers.

Essential oils today are generally extracted in one of four ways. Citrus seed extracts are generally made through cold-pressing. This means that the seeds are chopped and pressed, resulting in watery oil that has a shorter shelf-life than most essential oils, generally 6-8 months.

Many oils are made using solvent extraction, where the plant is mixed with a solvent. The solution distilled into a concentrated resin, which is combined with alcohol. The alcohol is allowed to evaporate, leaving behind the pure essential oil. When possible, avoid using oils extracted by this method. The solvents used often leave behind chemical traces of themselves, which can trigger reactions in people and animals, ranging from hives to allergies to headaches, and even depress the immune system.

Most aromatherapists prefer to use oils extracted through steam distillation: no residues are left behind in this process, and they are considered more pure. Steam distillation extracts the essential oil in a still using pressurized steam. The steam carries the essential oils into a cooling pipe, where the vapors condense and the pure essential oils separate from the water.

The newest method of oil extraction is carbon dioxide extraction, which is quickly gaining popularity due to its simplicity and ability to produce pure, untainted essential oils. The plant is pressurized and turned into a liquid. When the chamber is depressurized, the carbon dioxide becomes a gas, leaving behind nothing but the pure essential oil. This method results in the most costly oils, though prices are slowly decreasing as more aromatherapists demand pure oils.

When choosing your oils, remember that animals are more sensitive to scents and chemicals than most humans. Choose the carrier oil that best suits its application. Take the time to find the best oils for your situation. The following chapter listing oils and their uses is but a taste of the many oils available today on the market. There are many fantastic books available with more information on essential oils and aromatherapy; some of them can be found at the end of this book in our bibliography. Research, experiment, and enjoy!

CHAPTER FOUR

Horse Scents:

Essential Oils for the Barn

"Horse sense is the thing a horse has which keeps it from betting on people."

~ W.C. Fields

Basil

Ocicum basilicum

Basil is a tonifying carminative, and works wonders on viruses and nerve disorders. It can be used to treat liver, kidney and urinary tract problems, as well as to instill feelings of calmness and warmth.

Benzoin

Styrax benzoin

With its sweet vanilla odor, benzoin has a calming, relaxing effect. It has antiseptic properties which make it useful in prolonging the life of other oils and salves: add one drop to every aromatherapy formula to lengthen shelf-life.

Benzoin increases circulation, making it useful in the treatment of aches and pains. It is also a natural skin conditioner: this combined with its antiseptic and anti-inflammatory properties make it a natural addition to any wound dressing.

Calendula

Calendula Officinalis

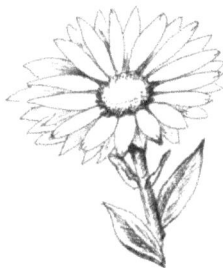

Calendula is a marvelous herb to prepare as an infused oil. It's gentle, calming and drawing nature will benefit any skin condition, from skin allergies and rashes, to dryness, bites and bruises.

Chamomile, German

Matricaria chamomilla

Similar to the herb, German chamomile oil has strong anti-inflammatory and anodyne properties, and will benefit all manner of aches and pains, including headaches and menstrual cramps. Apply a drop directly to swollen insect bites twice a day to reduce the pain.

Fennel

Foeniculum vulgare

Fennel oil is used to treat bloating and urinary disorders, as well as to heal bruises. When trying to slim down an overweight horse, consider using fennel aromatherapy, or adding a few seeds to the horse's feed – Fennel is a mild appetite suppressant.

Geranium, Rose

Pelargonium graveolens

Rose Geranium is unparalleled as a skin conditioner, with the possible exception of Myrhh, preferred by the ancient Greeks. Geranium oil can be used to treat wounds, burns, scars, bites, inflammations and infections. As geranium is planted in window boxes in Southern France to discourage mosquitoes and other biting insects, so may the essential oil be used to discourage bugs from bothering your horse.

In small amounts, its scent is calming to horses, and a drop on the skin can be used to relax a nervous horse.

Lavender

Lavandula angustifolia

Lavender is widely-known for its calming, soothing nature. Used topically, lavender is not only a calming scent, but also an anti-inflammatory that will soothe aching joints and muscles. This combined with its antiseptic properties makes lavender a natural remedy for wounds, insect bites, rashes and burns; Add a couple drops every day to wound dressings to insure proper healing.

In Europe, lavender was one of the four herbs used in the famous "Four Thieves Vinegar," so named for four men who tended the plague-afflicted for years without ever getting infected. They attributed their hardiness to the vinegar: every day before going out, the "four thieves" would drink a dram of the herb-infused vinegar, and wash their hands and faces in it upon returning home from the beds of the sick.

Lemon Eucalyptus

Eucalyptus citriodora

Lemon eucalyptus is anti-inflammatory and anti-bacterial, which makes it a fabulous ingredient in any salve destined to treat minor wounds and bruises. Combined with rose geranium and calendula, it will also help keep away biting insects.

Mugwort

Artemisia vulgaris

In Chinese medicine mugwort has long been used to alleviate bruises and swelling. The Native Americans burned it to purify spaces, similar to sage, and used it as a decoction for all manner of fevers and wounds. Externally, a mugwort infused oil can be applied to great effect in the treatment of sore muscles or skin infections.

Myrrh

Commiphora myrrha

Myrrh is arguably one of the most blessed oils: given to Jesus, used to mummify the dead in Egypt and as a wound dressing in Ancient Greece by the Olympiads, myrrh has a grand history. It is a luxurious treatment for any skin problem, including saddle sores, minor wounds and bites, and dry, cracking skin. It will close and speed the healing of most wounds when used topically: make sure that wounds are clean before applying myrrh. Added to tooth pastes or powders, it will benefit gums and teeth, alleviating soreness and acting as an antiseptic.

Opopanax

Illicium verum

The woody, musty scent of opopanax is, happily, also a flea and tick deterrant. Add a few drops in with your daily fly spray bottle, shake well before use, and spray away – knowing your horse is now much less likely to be a feast for deer ticks.

Rosemary

Rosemarinus officinalis

Any salve destined to treat inflammation and soreness simply *must* contain rosemary! Rosemary will produce a powerful liniment, heating and penetrating sore muscles and improving sluggish circulation. It will increase a horse's energy, alertness and memory, and a drop on the saddle can be a good aid for training.

Sage

Salvia officinalis

Sage oil is both antioxidant and antiseptic. The Native American Indians used it to stimulate hair growth.

For horses, it is a useful therapy for saddle sores and other areas where the hair has been rubbed off, as well as thinning tails accompanied by flaking skin, often a sign of a minor fungal infection.

Caution: Sage oil may reduce lactation in nursing mares.

Sandalwood

Santalum album

Sandlewood has a gentle, peaceful scent, and is

wonderful for treating inflammation, soreness and nerve problems – both due to its anti-inflammatory properties and the scent's ability to calm and relax both horse and rider.

Tea Tree
Melaleuca alternifolia

A member of the large and diverse eucalyptus family, tea tree is a strong antiseptic and anti-fungal oil. Use it to treat any minor wound, bite or skin infection.

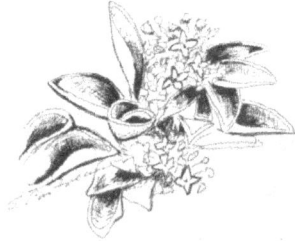

Though it has a powerful scent, tea tree is one of the few essential oils that is safe to put directly on the skin, undiluted. Used this way, it can rubbed onto insect bites to relieve itching and swelling, as well as applied to minor wounds to speed healing and deter infection.

Thyme

Thymus vulgaris

Similar to the dried herb, thyme oil is used in liniments and salves to treat sore, tired muscles. Combined with rosemary, thyme oil will produce a potent anti-inflammatory liniment.

Yarrow

Achillea millefolium

Yarrow-infused oil, particularly when combined with geranium or myrrh, is a wonderful balm for skin wounds and rashes, and can calm all manner of aggrieved skin.

Ylang-ylang

Cananga odorata

Known in the Far East for its ability to stimulate the growth of luxurious hair, ylang-ylang has been proven in western trials to control the production of scalp sebum, which is often a factor in slow hair growth, and even hair loss.

This oil can be used to great effect as an ingredient in any hair tonic or conditioner for horses.

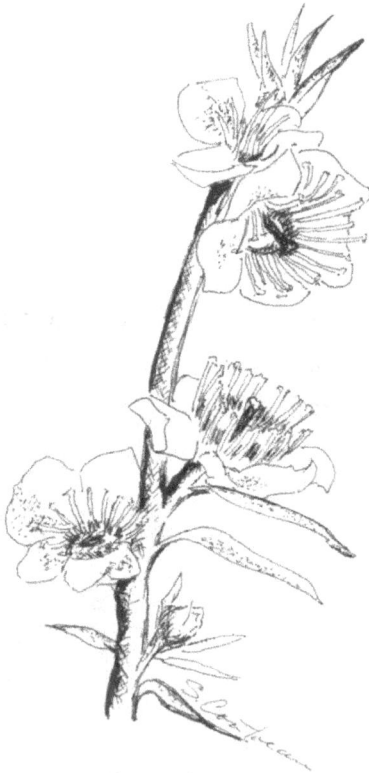

CHAPTER FIVE

How to Prepare Your Herbs

"Let a man decide upon his favorite animal and make a study of it. Let him learn to understand its sounds and motions. The animals want to communicate with man. But Wakan-Tanka does not intend that they should do so directly. Man must do the greater part in securing an understanding." ~ Brave Buffalo, Lakota Sioux Holyman, Standing Rock Reservation

Herbs are wonderfully beneficial to horses in their natural form, dried or fresh, mixed with grains or fed right from the hand. One sometimes wonders if any other method of application is even needed -- until the need arises.

There comes a day in almost every horse's life when she would benefit greatly from her owner lovingly applying a salve or poultice to an external bruise or wound. Braces can be used daily as a mild form of healing, or just as a reward for a horse's hard work on the trail. A chamomile infusion added to a drinking trough can calm nervous pasture-mates. And a picky eater not interested in your herbal offerings may respond to a tablespoon of herbal tincture added to his water. This chapter will teach you when and how to make these herbal remedies, and more.

INFUSIONS:

Most of us have enjoyed a warm cup of herbal tea at one time or another. In Europe, and among herbalists, the word for this beverage is an "infusion," warm water infused with the taste and benefits of an herb through the steeping process. Infusions are probably the easiest herbal remedy to make and enjoy. All you need is water, fresh or dried herbs, a kettle, and a heat source.

To make an herbal infusion, bring your water to a boil, and remove from the heat source. Add one tablespoon of dried herbs, or three tablespoons of fresh herbs, per cup of hot water. Cover and let steep for 10 to 15 minutes. (The longer it steeps, the stronger it will be. Dried roots can steep a bit longer, 15 to 20 minutes.) Strain the liquid through a cheesecloth and store in the refrigerator for 3-5 days.

Now that you've made an infusion, how can

you use it? Infusions carry the same properties as their herbal sires. They are, literally, waters that have been infused with the essential oils, nutrients, active compounds, and aromatics that the herb itself contained. A cup of an infusion can be added to your horse's drinking water for a mild effect, or may be tube-fed to a weakened, dehydrated horse for a rejuvenating effect. It can also be added to a warm hoof-soak to help draw out infections or relieve soreness. Or, try adding an infusion to the bucket of your horse's rinse water after his bath. A rosemary infusion will add shine and luster to his hair, as well as invigorate his joints and muscles.

BRACE:

In equine terms, a brace is a an invigorating liquid that is strong enough to be used to wash down one's horse after a hard ride, yet gentle enough to be used in bandages to focus on a particular sprain or minor wound. A brace can be as simple as a strong infusion with enlivening herbal properties, or more complicated: a half-teaspoon of your favorite tincture added to a cup of witch hazel. The combinations are endless, and with a bit of experimentation you will find what best suits you and your horse's needs.

POULTICES:

Poultices have been used in equine care for centuries to draw out infections and speed healing in traumatized areas. You can make a poultice out of any fresh or dried herb. Bring a pot of water to a full boil (for wound treatments, boil for 15 minutes to kill bacteria in the water) and add some of the hot water to the herbs, soaking them until they are softened. Strain the herbs, saving the infused liquid for a brace for later treatment or to add to the horse's water, depending on what herbs you are using. When the soaked herbs are near body-temperature, they are safe to put directly on the affected area. Use a clean cloth bandage to keep the poultice in place.

A fine example of an herbal poultice is yarrow, which will staunch bleeding, cleanse the wound and hasten healing. The infused water can also be added to your horse's drinking water to help heal the wound from the inside out.

TINCTURES:

Herbal tinctures are cold infusions of herbs that generally take two – six weeks to steep. They are generally made with high-proof alcohol such as brandy or vodka, apple cider vinegar, or glycerin. For equine use, we recommend making tinctures with apple cider vinegar, which is more palatable and benefits their digestive system. A tincture made with vinegar can be stored for up to 18 months. Having a few tried and true remedies on hand in tincture form can save you precious time in an emergency, when you can add a dropper of the tincture to drinking water or a poultice, rather than spending thirty minutes to boil water and steep herbs.

The procedure to prepare a tincture is very simple. In a glass jar, add one cup of dried herbs and cover with apple cider vinegar. Close the jar and store in a cool, dark place for two to six weeks. The longer it infuses, the stronger the tincture will be. When it is ready, strain off the liquid and store in a cool, dark place for up to 18 months. 15-30 drops of a tincture is considered equivalent to one cup of a fresh herbal infusion, again depending on the strength of your infusion.

INFUSED OILS:

Infused oils can be used directly on your horse for massage therapy, added to custom salves, and even used to condition your saddle and other leather tack.

There are several ways to infuse carrier oils. Both fresh and dried herbs may be used, although we prefer to use dried herbs. Fresh herbs have a higher water content than dried herbs, and the water can mix into the oil, which may shorten an oil's shelf life. When using fresh herbs, always make sure that they are washed clean and fully dried off before you infuse them.

The fastest way to infuse an oil is by heating the oil and herbs over the lowest heat on your stove for twenty minutes. The warmth allows the herbal properties to seep into the oil quite quickly, making this an efficient method. However, heat also accelerates the breakdown process of oils, which can shorten their shelf life. When using this method, be sure you are using very stable oils, such as canola or apricot oil. Olive oil is not suitable for heat infusion if you are planning on storing it for more than a week. The life of any infused oil can be prolonged by adding one-half teaspoon of vitamin E per cup of oil.

A gentler way to infuse oils through warmth is to place the herbs in a glass jar and cover them with oil, close the lid and place in a a sunny place outside or in a window for 1-7 days. This works quite well. Strain off the oil when it has reached its desired strength and use as desired. However, keep in mind that oils which are prone to spoilage are better off not being exposed to sunlight, and will not last quite as long after they have been heated in this manner.

Cold-infusion poses the least amount of stress to your carrier oil, and is easy to perform. Again, simply place the herbs is a glass jar, cover, and place in a dark cupboard at room temperature for 2-6 weeks. When the herbal infusion has reached the strength you desire, strain and store.

SALVES:

A salve is a wax and oil based ointment that is great for spot treatments. Salves have been used throughout history to condition the hair and skin, heal wounds and treat skin ailments. Solid and long-lasting, a salve is a convenien way to take herbal remedies on the road. In medieval times, wives would often make up a salve for their husbands to take into battle or on long voyages.

Salves are relatively easy to make. You can use fresh or dried herbs, or essential oils, or all three in your salves. The simplest way to make a salve is to heat one part shaved beeswax in four parts carrier oil on the stove or in a microwave, just enough to melt the beeswax. The wax will melt best if you cut it into small pieces or use beeswax beads. Remove the mixture for the heat and stir it a few times. If you are using an herb-infused carrier oil, then your job is done. If you are adding essential oils to the mixture, add them now and stir again. Now pour the mixture into a suitable container and let cool. It will harden as it cools, and store for 12-18 months, depending on what kind of oils you use. Adding a drop of benzoin essential oil or the oil from a 400 IU vitamin E oil capsule for every 4 ounces of salve will also prolong your salve's shelf life.

CHAPTER SIX

Rescue Recipes

*"There is no secret so close as that between a rider
and his horse."*

~Robert Smith Surtees

Here are a number of special things you can create for your horses' comfort and to further explore your passion for herbs. Each of our time-honored recipes has been extensively tested and developed under natural conditions to bring soothing comfort. These have been thoroughly tested on our own animals, as well as used by fellow equestrians and friends for therapeutic benefits.

Most herbal remedies, like these, made without preservatives should be used within a week or two, and kept refrigerated. The pleasure also comes from making them over and over again.

Always begin in clean, sterile surroundings and first sterilize all of your utensils and receptacles.

Remember to label and date each finished product, so you can keep track of its shelf life. It is beneficial to keep a journal of your herbal creations to note what works best, and where you might want to make changes.

Many of us also use Reiki Healing on all foods and formulas that we create, as this enhances purity and efficacy. If you are not Reiki trained you can still work in a climate of love and happiness, giving your work the best of your energies.

Fly & Flea Spritzer ~ an essential horse scent for barn & field

    1 Cup of purified water

    1 drop lemongrass essential oil

    1 drop pennyroyal essential oil

    1 drop lavender essential oil

    2 drops sage essential oil

Measure this into a sterile 8-ounce spray bottle with a tight cap. Use this generously, as needed. Just shake and spray!

This spritzer is a pleasure to make and should be used often. Spray carefully around the animal's muzzle & eyes & tail, as well as on harness & tack. As the horse flicks her tail, she disperses the good essence of this 'horse scent' around.

Citrus Flea Spritzer ~ so soothing in the heat of summer!

Simmer several orange, lemon or lime peels in 2 cups of water for 15 minutes – make sure to use a stainless steel or glass pot. Strain and cool. Pour carefully into your spray bottle; label & date.

Shake and Spray!

A Tick & Flea Spray for all seasons

1 Cup of Water

3 drops Palmarosa essential oil

3 drops Opopanax essential oil

Measure this into a sterile 8-ounce spray bottle, shake and spray.

Anti-tick Water
Add one dropper or ¼ tsp of Neem Extract to your horse's water daily.

Edible Anti-tick Powder

1 oz. cloves powder

1 oz. neem leaves

This can act like a systemic insecticide with beneficial results for your animal. Grind the ingredients together and add 1 tsp to feed daily.

Sleep-Safe Bedding

To repel insects in your horse's bedding, sprinkle one cup dried Chamomile and Pennyroyal in bedding in stall.

Note: Not recommended around pregnant mares.

Rosemary & Nettle Brace

Add 1 oz. dried or 3 oz. fresh stinging nettle leaves to 1 quart of boiling water. Remove from heat, cover and steep for 13 minutes.

Let cool and use as a brace to relieve muscle fatigue or add to your horse's wash water to condition hair.

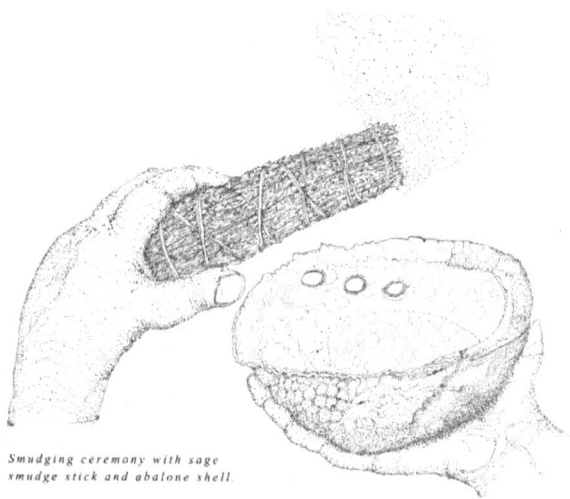

Smudging ceremony with sage smudge stick and abalone shell.

Smoke Them Out! (a natural flea bomb for the home)

Sometimes we bring the bugs from the barn and trail home with us. Use a bit of dried Elecampagne (*inula helenium*), also known as Horseheal, or its cousin Fleabane (I*nula dysenterica*) as an incense in flea-ridden areas instead of a smoke-bomb. This method is known as smudging by Native Americans, who used Sage and Cedar to banish pests.

In a fire-safe vessel, such as a ceramic bowl, light the herbs and then extinguish the flames. Fan the embers gently to keep them smoking and walk around your home, wafting smoke throughout the affected area. The smoke's scent effectively repels and discourages fleas.

Caution: This method is not recommended for use in a barn, where abundant hay makes fire prevention a top priority – barn fires are *not* a recommended method of flea eradication.

Fast Pain Relief Massage Oil

8 oz. Grapeseed Oil

10 Rosemary essential oil

10 drops Lavender essential oil

5 drops Lemon Eucalyptus essential oil

3 drops Thyme essential oil

3 drops Chamomile essential oil
1 drop Benzoin essential oil

This oil may rubbed into sore muscles and joints to quickly relieve aches and pains, whether from injuries or arthritis. Keep on hand in the barn for use after long, hard rides; this can be used on both you and your horse.

Hydration H$_2$O

The ingredients for this recipe are easy to find and should be kept on hand for emergencies in every barn. Use in cases of dehydration and electrolyte loss.

2 cups of Boiling Water

2 cups of Honey

½ Cup of Sea Salt

1 Gallon of Water

Bring the 2 cups of water to a boil, lower heat, and dissolve the honey and sea salt in the boiling water. Add solution to a gallon of water. Allow your horse to drink 1 cup every half hour.

Recovery Tea

This is a recipe for any tired horse, particularly older horses, studs, and horses under stress or recovering from illness.

In a covered pot, gently simmer one teaspoon of dried Korean ginseng root in one quart of water for 10 minutes. Remove from heat and steep another 20 minutes. Add one cup to your horse's water every day for two weeks at a time for noticeable difference.

> Note: Not recommended around pregnant mares.

R & R Supplement

1 /2 pound dried Chamomile

1/4 pound dried Red Clover

1/4 pound dried Chaparral

3 tablespoons daily in the feed may calm an over-spirited horse. This is also useful for horses on stall-rest, particularly with the anodyne properties of Chamomile.

Pregnanc-ease Feed

1 pound dried red raspberry leaves

1 pound dried stinging nettle leaves

Add three tablespoons to your pregnant mare's feed daily throughout her pregnancy to strengthen her urinary muscles and ensure proper fetal nutrition.

A nice brace for bathing can also be made out of nettles in the later days of your mare's pregnancy to relieve an aching back and give a nice shine to her coat.

Foaling Feed

½ pound dried stinging nettle leaves

½ pound dried chamomile flowers

½ pound dried marshmallow root

This mixture is recommended for mares after they have given birth to encourage proper milk production, ease post-partum discomfort and return the uterus to its original condition, as well as provide nutrients important for a young horse's development. Add two tablespoons daily to your mare's feed once she has given birth, for two to three weeks.

Horse Be Calm Perfume Oil

2 oz. Jojoba Oil

3 drops Lavender essential oil

2 drops Marjarom essential oil

2 drops Ylang Ylag essential oil

2 drops Sandlewood essential oil

Some horses need more assurance than others. This is a fantastic scent to wear around a new or jittery horse to help give it a sense of peace and calm. Trail riders seeking to take a bit of the edge off of their horse may want to wear this perfume, or even stroke a bit of it on their horse's mane.

Healing Salve

4 oz. Yarrow-infused Grapeseed oil

1 oz. Beeswax

5 drops Myrrh essential oil

10 drops Lavender essential oil

5 drops Tea Tree essential oil
1 drop Lemon Eucalyptus essential oil

This antiseptic, anti-bacterial salve is also an anodyne that can be applied to minor wounds, bruises and insect bites to speed healing. In lieu of a pre-made salve, any or all of these same essential oils can be added to aloe vera juice or gel, which is itself a cooling anti-bacterial.

Hair and Hoof Formula

4 oz. Horsetail

4 oz. Calendula

2 oz. Stinging Nettle

2 oz. Kelp

2 oz. Dandelion

Mix the dried herbs together and add 3 Tbs. to your horse's feed daily to improve coat and hooves.

Ear Cleanser

2 oz. Witch Hazel

1 oz. Aloe Vera Juice

5 drops Lavender essential oil

3 drops Geranium essential oil

Using a clean cotton pad or gauze, clean the ears with a small amount of this lotion for ear wax, mites, and scales. Store in the refrigerator.

Manageable Mane Base

1/2 Gallon Apple Cider Vinegar

1/2 cup rosemary

1/2 cup calendula petals

1/4 cup horsetail

Place the herbs in a large glass container and add the vinegar. Close and store in cool, dark place for two to four weeks. Label and store in a cool, dark place for up to 18 months. One cup of this vinegar can be added to a gallon of water for a refreshing, hair-conditioning brace and to help alleviate skin allergies.

Manageable Mane Shampoo

6 oz. Water

4 oz. Glycerin

2 oz. Manageable Mane Base

Mix ingredients and use as a refreshing, foaming shampoo.

Optional EssentialOils:

To discourage fleas and insects, add 5 drops Tea Tree or Geranium

To encourage hair growth, add 5 drops Cedar or Ylang-Ylang

To bring out highlights, add 5 drops Chamomile

To darken hair, add 5 drops Sage.

Anti-fungal Hoof Conditioner

2 oz. Avocado or Jojoba oil

2 oz. Horsetail-infused Olive oil

5 drops Lemon essential oil

2 capsules vitamin E oil

Mix ingredients together and store for up to one year in a cool place. A small amount of this oil on a clean cloth or pad can be used to clean, restore shine and condition hooves.

Leather Tack Conditioner

½ cup lavender-infused apricot oil

2 tbs Jojoba oil

5 drops tea-tree essential oil

3 drops geranium

1 drop myrrh essential oil

This oil can be used alone to help condition and waterproof all your leather tack, or you can use it to make a salve which will further waterproof boots and more. It will help protect your leather from mold and rot, as well as keep away bugs.

Remember, when oiling your tack a little goes a long way. Apply a small amount to a small cloth and rub it into your new tack, or any tack that needs a bit revitalizing. Oils may darken your tack, so in some cases it is best to apply the oil to the underside of the leather only.

CHAPTER SEVEN

Ailments & Remedies: A Table

Ailment	Internal Herbs	External Herbs	Oils
Aging	Bilberry, Cleavers, Red Clover, Dandelion, Ginseng, Hawthorn, Milk Thistle		Geranium, Rosemary, Thyme
Allergies	Chamomile, Dandelion, Elecampane, Garlic, Goldenrod, Marshmallow, Mullein, Nettles	Calendula Yarrow	Yarrow

Anxiety	Borage, Chamomile, Red Clover, Mullein	Yarrow & Willow	Basil, Benzoin, Geranium, Lavender, Sandlewood
Appetite	Devil's Claw, Garlic, Goldenrod, Kelp, Marshmallow, Milk Thistle, Nettles, Peppermint		Fennel, Rosemary
Arthritis	Borage, Burdock, Chamomile, Cleavers, Comfrey leaves, Dandelion, Devil's Claw, Hawthorn, Marshmallow, Meadowsweet Nettles, Thyme, Willow	Nettles, Peppermint, Thyme Comfrey leaves Meadowsweet & Nettles	Benzoin, Thyme, Chamomile, Lavender, Mugwort, Rosemary, Sandlewood, Thyme
Blood Cleansing	Burdock, Red Clover, Dandelion, Echinacea, Garlic, Kelp,		Tea Tree, Yarrow

	Milk Thistle, Nettles, Yarrow		
Blood Pressure	Bilberry, Celery, Cleavers, Garlic, Hawthorn, Willow		Geranium, Lavender
Bones	Boneset, Kelp, Horsetail, Stinging Nettle, Comfrey Leaves, Horsetail	Boneset & Comfrey leaves	
Bruises	Borage, Cleavers, Devil's Claw, Marshmallow, Meadowsweet Nettles, Thyme, Willow	Calendula, Marshmallow, Nettles, Thyme, Willow bark	Calendula, Fennel, Lavender, Myrhh, Rosemary, Sandlewood, Thyme
Cancer	Chaparral, Cleavers, Red Clover, Dandelion, Garlic,	Chaparral, Cleavers, Red Clover, Garlic, Plantain	Tea Tree

	Ginseng, Milk Thistle, Plantain, Yarrow	Burdock, Willow, Yarrow	
Circulation	Cleavers, Garlic, Hawthorn, Meadowsweet Nettles	Nettles & Willow, Mint	Benzoin, Rosemary
Colic	Apples, Bilberry, Boneset, Chamomile, Cleavers, Goldenrod, Kelp, Marshmallow, Milk Thistle, Peppermint, Willow		Basil, Fennel
Conges-tion	Red Clover, Elecampane, Garlic, Marshmallow, Mullein, Nettles, Thyme	Thyme, Mint	Lemon Eucalyptus

Constipa-tion	Apples, Boneset, Cleavers, Marshmallow		
Coughing	Borage, Burdock, Comfrey Leaves, Marshmallow, Mullein		
Dehydra-tion	Kelp, Marshmallow, Nettles	Burdock & Willow	
Depress-ion	Borage, Chaste Tree, Ginseng, Peppermint		Basil, Geranium, L. Eucalyptus, Rosemary
Detoxifica tion	Burdock, Dandelion, Garlic, Nettles, Yarrow		Basil
Diarrhea	Apples, Bilberry, Marshmallow		
Digestion	Chamomile, Comfrey Leaves, Dandelion,		Basil, Fennel, Rosemary

	Goldenrod, Peppermint Marshmallow, Nettles,		
Ears	Garlic, Mullein	Calendula, Mullein Flowers	Yarrow
Eyes	Bilberry, Marshmallow	Bilberry	
Fatigue	Elecampane, Ginseng, Peppermint, Thyme, Yarrow	Peppermint, Rosemary	Lemon Eucalyptus, Rosemary,
Fear	Chamomile, Echinacea, Mullein	Yarrow	Basil, Benzoin, Chamomile, Sandlewood
Fever	Boneset, Borage, Burdock, Chaparral, Garlic, Ginseng, Meadowsweet Peppermint, Willow, Yarrow	Peppermint	Yarrow

Fertility	Chamomile, Chaste Tree, Kelp, Nettles, Thyme, Yarrow		Chamomile, Yarrow
Fleas	Garlic	Calendula, Garlic, Mint, Thyme, Yarrow	Chamomile, Geranium, Opopanax
Flies	Garlic	Calendula, Yarrow, Peppermint	Geranium, Lemon Eucalyptus, Opopanax
Hair Care	Horsetail, Kelp, Marshmallow, Nettles	Calendula, Horsetail, Marshmallow, Nettles, Plantain	Geranium, Lavender, Rosemary, Sandlewood, Tea Tree, Ylang-Ylang
Hair Growth	Horsetail, Kelp, Nettles	Burdock, Nettles, Peppermint	Geranium, Rosemary, Sage, Ylang-Ylang
Heart	Elecampane, Hawthorn, Meadowsweet, Willow		Benzoin, Rosemary, Sandlewood
Hooves	Cleavers, Calendula,	Garlic, Horsetail,	Calendula, Geranium,

	Horsetail, Kelp, Marshmallow, Nettles	Willow, Yarrow, Plantain, Meadowsweet	Myrhh, Rosemary, Tea Tree
Hormone & Glands	Boneset, Borage, Chaste Tree, Red Clover		Fennel
Immune System	Boneset, Echinacea, Garlic, Ginseng	Elecampane, Willow, Thyme	Lavender
Inflamma-tion	Boneset, Borage, Chamomile, Cleavers, Devil's Claw, Marshmallow, Meadowsweet Nettles, Thyme, Willow	Nettles, Thyme, Cleavers, Celery, Boneset	Chamomile, Lavender, Lemon Eucalyptus, Myrhh, Rosemary, Sandlewood, Thyme
Internal Bleeding	Horsetail, Raspberry Leaves, Yarrow		Yarrow
Joints	Boneset, Borage, Burdock,	Nettles, Peppermint,	Chamomile, Lavender, Rosemary,

	Chamomile, Dandelion, Devil's Claw, Hawthorn, Horsetail, Marshmallow, Meadowsweet, Nettles, Thyme, Willow	Thyme	Sandlewood, Thyme
Kidneys	Burdock, Dandelion, Goldenrod, Horsetail, Marshmallow, Yarrow		Basil, Yarrow
Laminitis	Dandelion, Garlic, Kelp, Marshmallow, Meadowsweet Nettles, Thyme, Willow	Nettles	Chamomile, Lavender, Myrhh, Rosemary, Sandlewood
Liver	Bilberry, Dandelion, Horsetail, Milk Thistle		Basil, Yarrow

Lyme Disease	Ginseng, Hawthorn, Meadowsweet Nettles, Thyme, Willow	Nettles, Peppermint, Thyme, Garlic, Kelp, Willow	Basil, Lavender, Rosemary, Sandlewood, Thyme
Minor Wounds & Bites	Calendula, Comfrey Leaves, Echinacea, Garlic, Goldenrod, Thyme, Yarrow	Bilberry, Calendula, Comfrey Leaves, Echinacea, Garlic, Goldenrod, Horsetail, Marshmallow, Plantain, Raspberry Leaves, Yarrow	Benzoin, Chamomile, Lavender, Lemon Eucalyptus, Myrhh, Sandlewood, Tea Tree, Yarrow
Navicular	Borage, Burdock, Chamomile, Comfrey Leaves, Devil's Claw, Hawthorn, Horsetail, Marshmallow, Meadowsweet Nettles, Thyme, Willow	Nettles, Peppermint	Chamomile, Lavender, Rosemary, Sandlewood, Thyme

Nervous	Chamomile, Mullein	Yarrow, Willow	Basil, Benzoin, Geranium, Lavender, Sandlewood
Nursing	Chamomile, Chaste Tree, Dandelion, Marshmallow, Milk Thistle, Nettles, Raspberry Leaves	Nettles	Chamomile, Fennel, Lavender
Nutrition	Red Clover, Kelp, Nettles, Raspberry Leaves		
Pain	Chamomile, Devil's Claw, Meadowsweet Thyme, Willow	Thyme, Boneset, Willow, Meadowsweet, Nettles	Benzoin, Chamomile, Lavender, Mugwort, Rosemary, Sandlewood

Pregnant Mares	Nettles, Raspberry Leaves	Nettles	
Respira-tory Tract	Borage, Chaparral, Comfrey Leaves, Elecampane, Marshmallow, Mullein, Nettles, Thyme		Lemon Eucalyptus
Skin Allergies & Rashes	Burdock, Calendula, Chaparral, Comfrey Leaves, Dandelion, Elecampane, Garlic, Horsetail, Marshmallow, Nettles, Yarrow	Borage, Burdock, Calendula, Chaparral, Cleavers, Horsetail, Marshmallow, Plantain, Yarrow	Calendula, Geranium, Lavender, Sage
Snake Bite	Echinacea, Garlic, Yarrow	Echinacea, Plantain, Yarrow	Lavender, Lemon Eucalyptus, Tea Tree

Ticks	Garlic	Garlic, Thyme, Peppermint, Yarrow	Basil, Chamomile, Geranium, Opopanax
Tonic	Burdock, Celery, Chaparral, Red Clover, Comfrey Leaves, Dandelion, Ginseng, Nettles, Yarrow		Basil, Rosemary, Yarrow
Urinary Tract	Celery, Cleavers, Dandelion, Goldenrod, Horsetail, Marshmallow, Plantain, Willow, Yarrow		Basil, Fennel,
Worms	Black Walnut, Clove, Elecampane, Garlic, Mullein, Thyme, Wormwood		Basil, Tea Tree, Thyme

CHAPTER EIGHT

Notable Herbal Cancer Treatments

"Nutrients are used in veterinary medicine both to support the cancer patient's energy needs and to serve as specific therapeutic tools." ~ Gregory K. Ogilvie, 1995; "Nutritional Approaches to Cancer Therapy," in Schoen, Allen M., MS, & Susan G. Wynn, DVM. *Complementary and Alternative Veterinary Medicine: Principles and practice.* 1998. NY: Mosby.

Herbs have always been recognized for their tasty, meal-enhancing properties. The success of secret family recipes all over the world hinge upon the proper combinations of herbs to tantalize and delight the palate. Now, scientists working with the U.S. Department of Agriculture have found that almost all household herbs also out-perform fruits, vegetables, and even garlic, when it comes to their antioxidant potential. Herbs are an abundant source of antioxidants and could provide potential anticancer benefits when supplementing a balanced diet.

147

Researchers ranked oregano, dill, thyme, rosemary and peppermint as having the highest amount antioxidant activity, with many other household spices and herbs following closely behind. Many of the highest ranked herbs, including oregano, contain *rosmarinic* acid, a strong phenol antioxidant. Oregano in particular was found to have 3 to 20 times higher antioxidant activity than the other herbs studied. Furthermore, oregano was found to be 12 times more powerful than oranges, and 42 times more than apples: eating one tablespoon of fresh oregano with a meal will reap the same benefits as consuming one apple – without the calories or sugars.

Antioxidants are important in the diet of all animals, reducing certain free radicals and the risk of cancer and heart disease. In this chapter, we will examine several herbal treatments for cancer, both new and old.

The story of Harry Hoxsey and his fight with the medical establishment over unorthodox cancer treatments is both fascinating medical drama and an important historical episode in the development of alternative medicine in the twentieth century.

~ Andrew Weil, Author of Spontaneous Healing

Hoxsey Anti-Cancer Formula & Treatments

This story begins with John Hoxsey, a horse farmer in Illinois, who found his Percheron stallion had a malignant tumor on its right hock in 1840. He could not bear to shoot the animal, so being a Quaker, he turned his prized horse out to pasture to die peacefully, yet observed him to make sure he was not suffering. He noticed the tumor had stabilized three weeks later, and watched the horse browsing deep in a profusion of weeds in a corner of the pasture, eating different plants not part of its normal diet.

Slowly the tumor shrank and dried up and within three months it separated from the healthy tissue and was removed. Hoxsey began to experiment with the various herbs revealed to him by "horse sense" along with other popular herbal remedies of the day. He became well known for treating animals with cancer and tumors and so a legend was born. He handed down his formulas through generations. His grandson John C. Hoxsey was a veterinarian in southern Illinois who first tried the cancer remedies successfully on people. "His son Harry showed an early interest and began working with him," says Kenny Ausubel, in his landmark book documenting the Hoxsey Cancer treatments.

149

"After his father's death, Harry founded the first Hoxsey Cancer Clinic in 1924."

Harry Hoxsey (1901-1974), a self-taught healer, cured many cancer patients using an herbal remedy for over three decades that was handed down by his great-grandfather. The charismatic practitioner of herbal folk medicine, born in Illinois, faced unrelenting opposition and harassment from a hostile medical establishment. Nevertheless, two federal courts upheld the "therapeutic value" of Hoxsey's internal tonic. The Hoxsey Cancer Clinic in Dallas was the world's largest private cancer center, by the 1950s, with branches in seventeen states.

It all began with horses. In this case, the Percheron stallion led his master to new herbal wisdom and the vitality to treat one of society's most dreaded disease. While this treatment continues for horses, humans also suffer exacting similar needs. The external Hoxsey mixture selectively destroys malignant tissue. The internal Hoxsey liquid mixture strengthens the immune system. Hoxsey believed his treatment allowed the body to create an environment in which healing and tumor destruction occurred.

The Hoxsey treatment involves two mixtures. One to be used externally applied directly to the skin and includes "a red paste containing antimony trisulfide, zinc chloride, and bloodroot and a yellow powder containing arsenic sulfide, sulfur and talc." The other is used internally and is "a liquid containing licorice, red clover, burdock root, stillingia root, barberry, Cascara, prickly ash bark, buckthorn bark and potassium iodide." While taking the Hoxsey formula, patients are also encouraged to restrict their diet, use immune stimulants such as vitamin C and adopt a positive mental outlook.

The types of cancers that respond best to these treatments include **melanoma, lymphoma,** and **external (skin) cancer.** The clinic's patient brochure includes case histories of patients successfully treated for **breast, cervical, colon, prostate,** and **lung cancers.**

Hoxsey Cancer Formula Ingredients:

Red Clover fresh-dried blossoms (*Trifolium pratense.*),

Chaparral fresh-dried leaf (*Larrea tridentata*),

Licorice fresh-dried root (*Glycyrrhiza glabra*),

Oregon Grape fresh-dried root (*Berberis nervosa*),

Burdock fresh-dried root (*Arctium lappa*),

Sarsaparilla fresh-dried root (*Smilax ornata*),

Echinacea fresh root (*Echinacea angustifolia*),

Prickly Ash fresh-dried bark (*Zanthoxylum americanum*).

* The Dietary Supplement Health and Education Act of 1994 permits and encourages providing scientific data to assist you in making healthcare decisions.

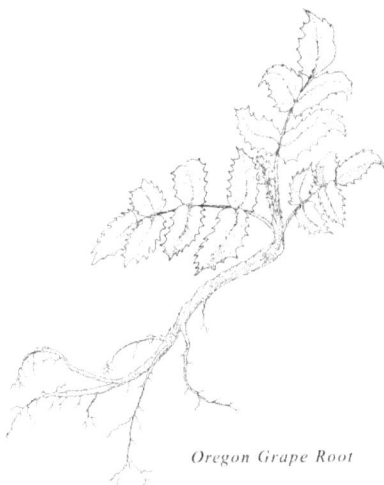

Oregon Grape Root

For additional information:

Hoxsey Clinic
Bio-Medical Center
PO Box 727
615 General Ferreira, Colonia Juarez
Tijuana, B.C. Mexico
Telephone: (011) 52-66-84-90-11

The University of Texas M. D. Anderson Cancer
Center
1515 Holcombe Boulevard
Houston, TX 77030
Telephone: (800) 392-1611
Web site:
www.mdanderson.org/departments/CIMER/

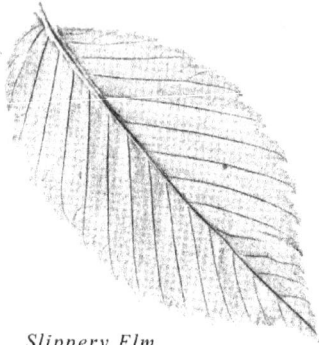

Slippery Elm

Cancer Support Formulas:
Essiac and Flor*Essence

"It is important to keep in mind that preparations such as the Ojibway tea (Essiac) were handed down from generation to generation for millennia through the oral tradition; if the tea hadn't been efficacious, it would have disappeared." ~ M. A. Richardson.

A Canadian oncology nurse, Rene Caisse who worked in a northern Ontario hospital in the 1920s, encountered an elderly patient whose breast cancer had been healed by an Ojibway medicine man 50 years earlier. She took careful note of the primary herbs used by the Ojibway Indians of Cobal, Ontario to make this tea. Sheep sorrel, burdock root, slippery elm bark, and Turkish rhubarb root are enhanced with the addition of watercress, red clover, kelp, and blessed thistle.

The original herbal formula was developed into a tonic promoted as a "cancer support formula" under the label of "Essiac" (her last name spelled backwards.) Over time and with experimentation the additional herbs were added

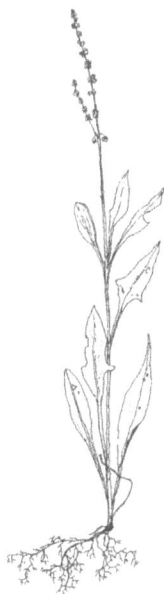

Sheep Sorrel

to this valuable formula to enhance its abilities to detoxify and it was named Flor*Essence. Dr. Charles Brusch and Elaine Alexander developed this latter formula in the 1970s out of special regard for Rene Caisse's successful 'ancient tonic'.

These important cancer support formulas have helped millions of people and animals in Canada and the United States throughout most of the twentieth century, and yet the legal and medical authorities in both countries persecuted the use of these products, as it did the Hoxsey cancer formulas. Both products are available, fortunately, across the country today from most herbal suppliers and health food stores, and are increasingly recognized by mainstream medicine.

Red Clover and Burdock are two plants most commonly shared in cleansing formulas, and "sheep sorrel is considered the most active herb for stimulating cellular regeneration, detoxification and cleansing," according to Rene Caisse and the doctors who worked with the original eight herb formula. The ingredients are: **burdock** root, *Arctium lappa,* **kelp,** *Laminaria digitata,* **blessed thistle** herb, *Cnicus benedictus,* **sheep sorrel,** *Rumex acetosella,* **slippery elm** bark, *Ulmus rubra,* **red clover** blossoms, *Trifolium pratense,* **Turkish rhubarb** root, *Rheum palmatum,* **watercress,** *Nasturtium officinale.*

"I am certain the remedy is efficacious... The sense of well being engendered in the patients is heartening and easily noticed ... The relief from pain is possibly the most dramatic change. In those cases of cutaneous cancer the evidence of quick healing and regeneration [is] visible and positive."
~ Dr. Charles Brusch, 1955, Brusch Medical Center in Cambridge, MA.

Absinthe: A New Anti-Cancer Remedy for Western Medicine?

Wormwood oil is used to flavor many foods and beverages. Many of us have tasted it in vermouth; a few of us may have even had the chance to try a true absinthe, which contains wormwood oil in large quantities. Absinthe was a popular alcoholic beverage in the late 1800s in Europe, but after being linked to several cases of brain damage, it was banned in most countries. Unfortunately, this has given wormwood a bad reputation – until recently.

In traditional herbalism, wormwood, or *Artemisia Absinthium*, was viewed as a powerful digestive treatment and known to remedy liver ailments. More recently, Chinese medicine has embraced *Artemisinin*, the active parent compound of the plant, to effectively treat cancer for the last 30 years in Vietnam and China.

Artemisinin is considered a very safe derivative of wormwood. The essential oil of wormwood contains the toxins *thujone* and *isothujone.* However, little of these are present in ordinary wormwood teas or tinctures.

Bioengineering professors at the University of Washington, Dr. Henry Lai and Dr. Narenda Singh, have recently conducted their own studies of wormwood, and believe it may be a safe alternative treatment for cancer patients. In their studies, *Artemisinin* eradicated breast-cancer cells and leukemia cells in less than 24 hours, while leaving virtually all normal breast cells and white blood cells unharmed.

Scientists believe *Artemisinin* works by creating free radicals when it interacts with iron. All cells need iron to replicate DNA every time they divide: all cancer cells have higher iron concentrations than healthy cells, generally 3 times as much in breast cancer cells, allowing them to divide and multiply at a much higher rate. By introducing more iron into cancer cells and then releasing *Artemisinin* into the system, the cancer cells are selectively eradicated. Theoretically, this raises high hopes for cancer patients, because the more acute the cancer, the higher the amounts of iron tend to be in the affected cells, so that the *Artemisinin* works even better in more severe cases.

This research has led to further studies. One laboratory study showed that many cultured cancer cells that did not respond to chemotherapy drugs were killed or contained by *Artemisinin*. At the University of Washington they have yet to find any type of cancer that will not respond to treatment *artemisinin*. Just five days after beginning the treatment, one of their laboratory studies cured a dog of a severe type of bone cancer, *osteosarcoma*, with the dog's massive tumor completely eradicated. In China, wormwood treatment has been reported to cure up to 60% of cancer cases, and stabilizing or remitting the rest.

Artemisinin treatment generally lasts for two years, as prolonged treatment ensures that the cancer does not return. While wormwood itself can cause nerve damage after prolonged, heavy use, its derivative *Artemisinin* is considered by scientists to be non-toxic, with little to no side-effects in the proper dosages.

"More than half of all cancer patients today will seek herbal remedies as part of their overall health support program. Most patients use these as an adjunct to their doctor's prescribed regimen of surgery, chemotherapy or radiation." ~ Complementary Cancer Therapeutics, 2003

Further Reading:

"The Ancient Herbal Tea that Became a Modern Cancer Tonic," in *The Doctors' Prescription for Healthy Living. Vol. 7 (8):* "Complementary Cancer Therapeutics." 2003.

Ausubel, Kenny. *When Healing Becomes a Crime: The Amazing Story of the Hoxsey Cancer Clinics and the Return of Alternative Therapies.* 2000. Rochester, VT: Healing Arts Press. 460-pages.

Richardson, M.A., et al. "Flor*Essence herbal tonic use in North America: a profile of general consumers and cancer patients." *HerbalGram* 2000(50): 40-46.

Schoen, Allen M. & Susan G. Wynn. *Complementary and Alternative Veterinary Medicine: Principles and practice.* 1998. NY: Mosby/Times Mirror. 820-pages.

CHAPTER NINE

Your Hands & Your Horse

"Now when the sun was setting, all those who had any that were sick with various diseases brought them to him; and he laid his hands on every one of them and healed them."   ~ Luke, 4:40

The healers of the East believe that all living beings have a vital life-force, or Chi, running through them. This energy is what animates the body. It runs its course through specific channels in the body, much as blood circulates to and from the heart, or our breath enters, flows through, and leaves our bodies at regular intervals. Chi energy runs through all organic things, including our horses.

It is now also believed by most western herbalists and naturopaths that energy does indeed run throughout our bodies along very specific pathways. Einstein's theories proved that our bodies are simply made of energy moving, or vibrating, at a particular level. When you manipulate this energy, you affect the body itself. The body's energy paths, known as *meridians*, pass through every part of our body. In fact, each body contains many meridians. The primary meridians govern the most basic organs. Just as blood flows on many different circuits and paths, from your heart to your kidneys to your fingers and toes, so do meridians.

Meridians teach us that no organ, no muscle, no bone nor tissue is an island. Everything in the body is interconnected and inter-dependent. Just as a misaligned spine can cause lower arm and leg pain, there is a spot on your horse's spine, which can benefit hindquarter ailments.

It has long been known in the medical community that various points on our body affect the functions of other corporeal areas. Studies linked to the National Institutes of Health have found that acupuncture dramatically relieves acute pain in 60 percent of the studies' patients –

that means that acupuncture really works. Placebo effects, or psychologically affected results, routinely benefit only one-third of test subjects.

Reflexology, acupressure, acupuncture and even phrenology, are all descendents of this belief. Modern energy healing practices, such as *Reiki, Hands On,* and *Hands of Light,* take these accepted practices even further using the healer's own hands to transmit or channel vital energy to the patient's body, following the meridians to sense and concentrate particularly on afflicted areas.

The point of this chapter is to familiarize you with your horse's body. We have included 13 diagrams in this chapter depicting equine physiology and major equine meridians. You do not have to be an energy healer or an acupressure specialist to lay your hands on your own horse. Today, equine massage is used in many stables to ease tension and muscle fatigue, increase the range of motion of your horse, and even speed healing. Try working a bit of gentle massage into your grooming routine. If you notice your horse has a particular problem, try the corresponding meridian points. At the very least, it will bring you closer to your horse.

"On horseback he seemed to require as many hands as a Hindu god, at least four for clutching the reins, and two more for patting the horse soothingly on the neck."
~Saki

Animal Body, Skeletal and Organ Diagrams

The anatomy of the horse is shown on the diagrams on page 89, including skeletal and muscular formations. These need to be well understood by any equine healing practitioner. For massage and acupressure therapists, direct work on or around specific muscles, joints, and organs will be conducted. As this type of therapy can result in significant pressure on parts of the body, only expert certified therapists should be allowed to conduct this therapy under the direction of a veterinarian. If working on your own horse, use a gentle touch and work slowly, watching your horse's reactions.

Energy bodywork, by contrast, is a non-invasive technique and only a feather-light touch, or no touch at all, is needed to bring about healing. After the chakras are balanced, the energy healer may then go directly to the part of the body diagnosed as injured or diseased. See the next section for a more detailed look at energy healing techniques.

Parts of the Horse

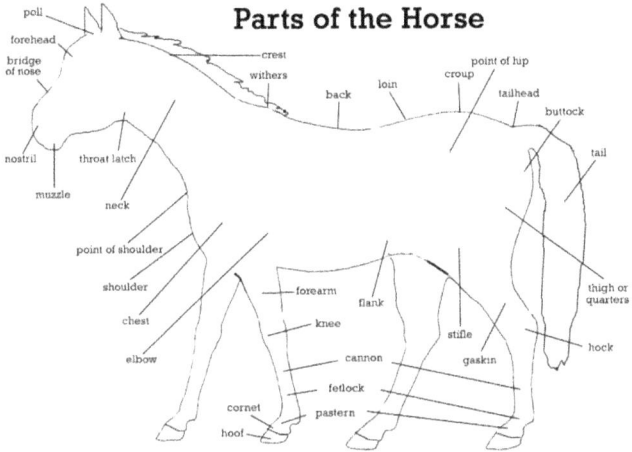

poll
forehead
crest
bridge of nose
withers
point of hip
croup
tailhead
back
loin
buttock
tail
nostril
throat latch
muzzle
neck
point of shoulder
shoulder
forearm
flank
chest
knee
stifle
thigh or quarters
elbow
cannon
gaskin
hock
fetlock
cornet
pastern
hoof

Organs of the Horse

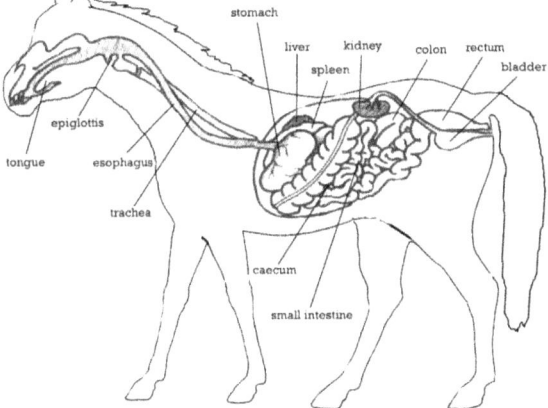

stomach
liver
kidney
colon
rectum
spleen
bladder
epiglottis
tongue
esophagus
trachea
caecum
small intestine

167

An Introduction to Equine Energy Healing

There appear to be so many methods of energy healing in today's literature. Which one works best? Which is the true way? We believe, as has been said for many hundreds of years in Zen philosophy, "all the ten thousand things are one". These words are entirely true concerning the art of energy healing. While there appear to be differences in techniques, in essence they are all the same.

As so many teachers have said over the years, including Carlos Castaneda and Deepak Chopra, a key factor in the power to heal is "intent". Chopra, in his *How to Know God: The Soul's Journey into the Mystery of Mysteries,* wrote "The act of creation is reducible to one ingredient: intention....There are no magic tricks to making a thought come true, no secrets in miracle-working. You just intend a thing and it happens". The simple focus of the healer's will with pure intent is the key to energy healing.

"…veterinarians are developing the ability to "listen" to horses to determine which part of the animal's gut hurts – the duodenum loop, the small or the large intestine."

~ Monty Roberts, The Man Who Listens to Horses, 1996.

Quieting the Mind

The most important step in obtaining pure intent is the quieting of the mind. There are many ways that work for quieting the mind. It is valuable to know these many ways, although they all get to the same end point. Sometimes, when our minds are particularly chaotic and filled with noise, we may have to try several of them until one that suits that day provides the necessary quiet.

Buddhism, Yoga, Transcendental Meditation, Tai Chi, and Qigong are all good methods taught throughout the United States that will help calm the mind. While these methods are directed at the concept of quieting the mind, focusing intent, and learning to direct energy flow, other activities can also lead many people down the right path. Jogging, rowing, skiing, carving, cooking and needlework, if done in a rhythmic balanced slow way can lead to an awareness of the circle of energy flow in our bodies, to our internal rhythm, and to how to direct our energy outward and pull the universal energy inward.

Gathering Energy to Heal

For many, visualization is an essential part of healing. The practice of Reiki involves the placing of hands side-by-side for a healing while visualizing ancient symbols said to be of Tibetan and Japanese origins, channeling healing energy. The Reiki practitioner assumes that the use of these symbols will always open up the channel for spiritual healing energy to be directed to the place of "dis-ease" in the patient's body. In Reiki, the hands are usually placed on, or slightly above the body, at the chakra points and along the body extremities, or above and below key joints, chakras, or trigger points. The hands are slightly cupped, like a swimmers', and the "bubbling well" in the center of the palm is slightly raised from touching the skin, while the thumb, digit finger, and three central fingers' tips are touching the body. Several levels of Reiki certification are available and many physical therapy and massage therapy professionals are now certified in Reiki and use it in hospitals and physician offices.

Healing Touch (also known as Therapeutic Touch) has similar side-by-side hand placements, but focuses on visualization of the energy flow and typically is done with the hands a small distance from the body. Also, in Healing Touch, there are other ways of placing hands at two separate chakra points, visualizing waves of energy between the hands, with the waves mixing like a whirlpool. Healing Touch was developed in the US several decades ago and has hundreds of thousands of health practitioners, with classes at medical schools for nurses and doctors. In the last decade, they have developed an important variation known as Healing Touch for Animals and reached out to train veterinarians, animal rescue workers, animal trainers, and pet owners. Several levels of Healing Touch certification are available, including the special certified training for animals healing.

About 2400 years ago, Lao Tzu, Chinese philosopher, wrote "The highest good is like water. Water gives life to the ten thousand things and does not strive." Healing energy flows from the healer like an artesian well, continuous sustenance of clear clean energy without worry about end... as it is channeled from our highest intent and is limitless.

Lakota Holy Man Black Elk said "you make of yourself a little hollow bone through which the energy flows." In other words, the energy worker is simply the conduit through which the universal healing energies flow to the source where the healing should take place. Animals are drawn to people in these relaxed, meditative states, and this is a primary way to "gentle" an over excited horse or nervous animal. With practice you will find that you transmit more than healing energy.

Techniques of Diagnosis

Diagnosis by the healing intuitive is done by various techniques. As part of the process, the healer relaxes the breath, clears the mind, and relinquishes judgement. Intuition will increase if we simply allow some of the limitations placed on our minds to be lifted. Don Juan Matus, the Mexican sorcerer who mentored Carlos Castaneda, stated, "The art of sorcerers is not really to choose, but to be subtle enough to acquiesce". Don Juan also taught, "as you chase away your internal dialogue, other items of awareness begin to fill in the empty space".

Some healing intuitives rely on their vision of energy fields, including chakras and auras. Such vision typically relies on indirect sight or sight through the third eye (located in the center of the forehead). Alan Watts, a scholar on Zen, in his "The Way of Zen" described that non-action seeing involved peripheral vision, wherein the eyes must be relaxed, not trying to see, and the mind must be calm, not grasping.

Barbara Ann Brennan in "Hands of Light" provides a number of exercises for enhancing the ability to see energy fields, or one's "clairvoyant vision". She suggests "gazing" at plants to see to see the greenish haze around their edge. Such a haze may look like heat waves or fog. For most of us, gazing at a living animal will enable us to see a grayish haze around the edge of the body. The more emotional or energized the animal, the larger this haze will become, and our chances of seeing color will be optimized.

Diagnosis also can be done through feeling differences in heat or energy through the palms of the hands. To sensitize your hands, you can hold your hands apart with the palms facing each other. Move the hands close together, about 3 inches apart, and then further away, about 12 inches apart, and feel the energy field as you move your hands back and forth in this distance range of 3 inches to 12 inches. It will feel like a pliable ball of energy that you can tangibly squeeze. Do the same in using your palms to feel the energy field around your head, holding your palms about two feet from your ears and moving them back and forth from that outside distance to about 6 inches away. At some point, you will feel the edge of your energy field, and will be able to practice expanding that field by pumping out your energy.

In the diagnosis of animals, the healing intuitive moves the palms of the hands from chakra to chakra, along the center of the body, and then along the extremities, giving special attention to all key joints. Generally heat is readily detectable in areas where pain or inflammation is occurring. Sometimes, in areas of tumors, cysts or other types of disease, the healing intuitive will feel a heaviness, denseness. Some will sense a darkness. Each intuitive is different. The key is to note the areas where there are marked differences – whether the differences are sensed as heat, cold, color, light, emotion, or density.

A precise diagnosis, for many healers, involves the use of a pendulum. Ideally, a clean clear crystal is hung from a short string or chain of about 6 inches. The pendulum is hung over each chakra to see whether it moves in a clockwise circle, a counter-clockwise circle, a straight swing, or not at all. Most healers experience that a clockwise circle denotes an open chakra and no movement or counterclockwise circles denote a closed movement. Blocked energy at any chakra is an indication of disease, either existing or pending. Distortion from a perfect circle, e.g., elliptical or straight-line movement, indicates emotional distortion. The wider the clockwise circle, the more open the chakra. Energy healing of the chakras should show immediate results in opening them up. The pendulum may be used both before and after healing.

Veterinarians in South Africa have experienced remarkable success in treating a wide spectrum of large and small animals using the pendulum. This is yet another ancient device for discerning areas special needs in modern situations, especially where time and money are deciding factors.

Techniques of Energy Clearing

To clear an energy field, the healing intuitive combs spread fingers through the energy field, about 4 to 6 inches from the animals body, and feels electrical prickling in the finger tips where there are problems. General healing involves continued raking until the energy field is finally cleared. The spread fingers grab onto bad, or blocked, energy as they move through the patient's energy field. At the end of the limb or body part being raked, the healer continues the raking about 12 inches from the body's end and then throws the raked negative energy away. The process continues... rake then discard, rake then discard. If some accumulated prickling or negative energy bothers the healer, the hands are usually shaken until everything is released.

Another method of throwing away the negative energy simply involves facing the palms outward and focusing on clean energy pouring out through the hands to the cleansing universe. The healer visualizes being an open channel, like a flexible open bamboo, though which the clean universal healing energy flows unimpeded.

Many healers say a prayer of protection before healing, asking for the highest purest spiritual forces of the universe to protect the patient and the healer during the healing process. The outcome of any healing should be what is best for the highest purpose of the spiritual life of the patient. Healers hand themselves over to the process, as channels for universal spirit to work for the good of the patient.

Techniques of Energy Healing and Balancing

Reiki and Healing Touch both focus on the chakra points. When Reiki is performed on a human, the healer starts from the crown chakra and moves down to the root chakra, and then addresses the limbs. In Healing Touch for

Animals, the healer starts at the root chakra and moves to the crown chakra, and then addresses the limbs. The hands are placed side by side, in a cupped manner, with the center of the palms above the chakra. After healing each chakra until the hand feels that that position is done, balancing of the chakras can be done by placing one hand on one chakra and another on the next, feeling the flow of energy between the chakra points.

After dealing with the chakra points and limbs, the healer intuitively addresses any location that the hands are taken to for special healing of a diseased organ or joint. Thereafter, the healing is finished by standing a couple of feet away and holding the hands to sense and heal the entire energy field of the patient's body, willing it to be balanced, clear, energized and protected.

Animal Chakra Points & Energy Meridians

The following diagrams provide the location of chakras, energy meridians and emergency pressure points for horses. Other animals have their points in similar locations. Animal chakra points are similar to those of people, except that the third, fifth, sixth, and seventh points are along the spine. The fourth point is in the center of the animal chest, below the base of the neck. The first two points are near each other, one on the animal forehead and the other at the top (crown) of the head. When working with a small animal, like a miniature dog, these points can be treated together, as the palm of the hand fits over both at one time.

When doing energy work on a horse, the work should begin at the last chakra point at the base of the tail and progress up to the first chakra point at the crown.

TTEAM Techniques

The **T**ellington **T**ouch **E**quine Awareness **M**ethod is a training system for horses that incorporates bodywork, ground, and riding exercises to help improve co-ordination, balance, and athletic ability. This also deepens the understanding between horse and rider. American horsewoman Linda Tellington-Jones developed it in the 1970s. TTEAM is used around the world now by competition and pleasure riders, veterinarians and trainers to educate and rehabilitate horses of all ages and breed types.

Inspired by the Feldenkrais method of Awareness Through Movement, "TTEAM techniques take horses through a variety of gentle exercises to help alter existing habitual postural patterns by encouraging them to use their body more effectively," says Sarah Fisher, a Certified TTEAM Practitioner. This gentle system of inspired touch and stroking also creates amazing bonds. It has proven so successful with horses that it is now applied to all domestic animals.

Equine Chakra Points

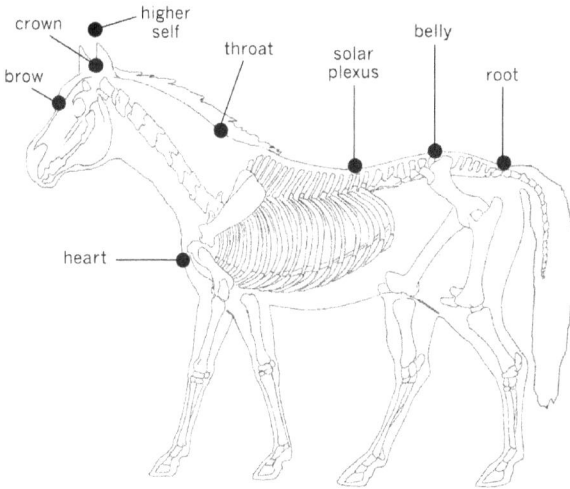

Root Chakra – Governs sex drive, reproductive organs, the legs and primal instincts.

Belly Chakra – Governs digestion and issues relating to family and self-confidence.

Solar Plexus Chakra – Governs the diaphragm, solar plexus and issues of safety, protection, and one's place in society.

Heart Chakra – Governs the heart, chest, and issues relating to forgiveness, love, stress and anger.

Throat Chakra – Governs the mouth, throat and respiratory system, as well as issues relating to voicing thoughts, speaking out.

Brow Chakra – Governs the eyes, nasal passages and issues of the conscious mind.

Crown Chakra – Governs the head and issues of the soul.

Higher Self Chakra – Connects the crown chakra with the higher self and the astral body. Allows one to access their higher purpose in life.

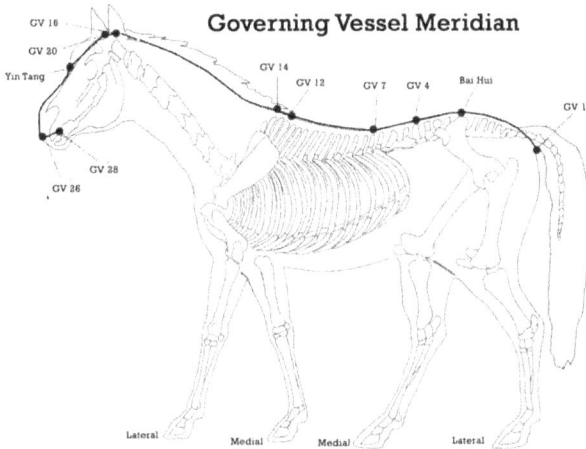

Governing Vessel Meridian

GV 16
GV 20
Yin Tang
GV 14
GV 12
GV 7
GV 4
Bai Hui
GV 1
GV 28
GV 26
Lateral   Medial   Medial   Lateral

GV 1   Regulates defecation, aids both constipation and diarrhea. Instigates newborns' first bowel movement.

GV 4   Strengthens lower back and urogenital tract. Aids intestinal

        disorders.

GV 12   Use after long illness to strengthen entire body.

GV 14   Stimulates immunity, eases heatstroke.

GV 26   Aids shock, seizures, heatstroke and collapse. Can also stimulate respiration in newborns.

Yin Tang   Calms horses. Aids colds and coughs.

Bai Hui   Major point for all hindquarter ailments.
           Aids heatstroke and overexertion.

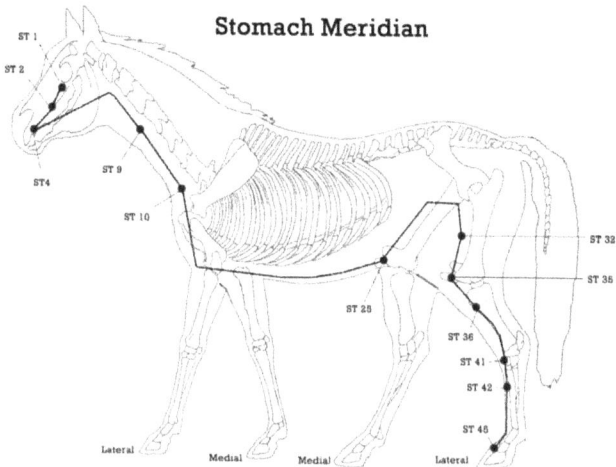

Stomach Meridian

ST 1
ST 2
ST4
ST 9
ST 10
ST 25
ST 32
ST 35
ST 36
ST 41
ST 42
ST 45
Lateral
Medial
Medial
Lateral

ST 1-4   Relieve facial problems, including paralysis, tensions and toothaches.

ST 2   Major pain relief and relaxation point for the entire body. Use with point ST 36 for colic.

ST 25   Relieves leg and abdominal problems. Boosts blood flow in the legs.

ST 35   Aids pain and arthritis in the stifle. Reduces pain in the hind leg joint.

ST 36   Main point for the gastrointestinal tract and the abdomen. Aids digestion and, used with ST 2, helps in colic problems. Builds the immune system and increases contractions during labor.

ST 41   Helps with hind leg lameness and soreness.

ST 45   Aids digestion, abdominal problems, and convulsions.

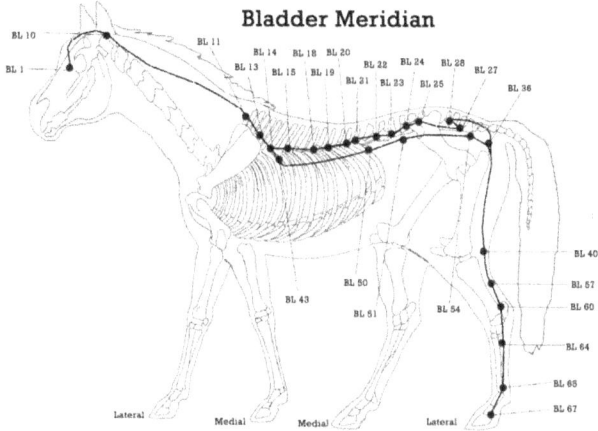

Bladder Meridian

BL 10   Aids cervical pain, also shoulder and back pain. May help wobblers.

BL 11   Aids any bone or joint problems, speeds bone healing. Relieves rheumatoid arthritis.

BL 13   Benefits all lung problems, including asthma.

BL 14   Calms horse, releases lung congestion.

BL 15   Calms horse, regulates energy flow.

BL 18   Aids all liver problems, relieves back pain and tendonitis.

BL 19   Helps liver and ligament problems.

BL 20   Relieves medial stifle disorder and aids
         digestion.

BL 21   Helps gastrointestinal and lateral stifle
         disorders.

BL 22   Treats thyroid, adrenal and lower back
         problems. Releases
         abdominal pain and swelling. Relieves
         colic, and detoxifies the
         liver, kidney and bladder.

BL 23   General point to relieve arthritis, and
         chronic lower back pain. Boosts Immune
         system.

BL 24   Energizes and moves stagnant energy.
         Aids lumbosacral
         problems.

BL 25   Relieves diarrhea and constipation, as
         well as hock, neck, shoulder, lower back
         and stifle pain.

BL 27   Aids digestion. Relieves sciatica and
         lower back problems.

BL 28   Benefits bladder disorders, and neck and
          back pain. Aids colic.

BL 40   Relieves pain and stiffness in hip, stifle
          and lower back.

BL 60   Use to relieve hock problems and soft
          tissue injuries.

BL 65   Benefits navicular, tendonitis and
          arthritis.

BL 67   Balances meridian energy. Aids all hoof
          problems and navicular.

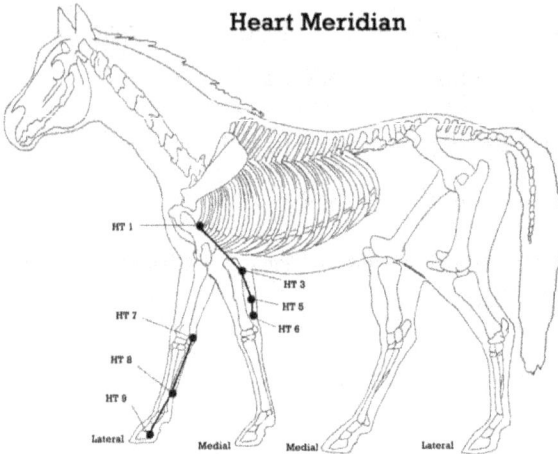

Heart Meridian

HT 1   Clears meridian energy flow. Relaxes horse and relieves shoulder arthritis

HT 5   Aids eyesight problems and forelimb stiffness.

HT 6   Aids behavioral problems and forelimb stiffness. Calming point.

HT 7   Major point for relaxing and centering horse mentally. Aids carpal joint problems.

HT 9   Balances meridian energy and alleviates fevers. Use in cardiovascular emergencies

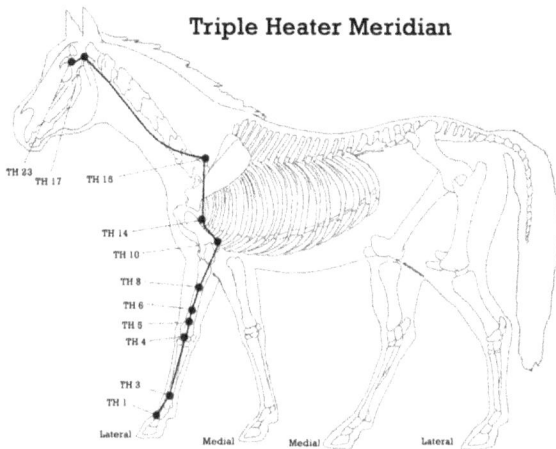

Triple Heater Meridian

TH 4   Aids pastern and tendons. Unblocks meridian. Benefits chronic conditions resulting from low kidney functioning.

TH 5   Eases navicular pain, rheumatism and tendonitis.

TH 6   Aids colic, navicular and neck problems.

TH 8   Releases shoulder, neck and forelimb.

TH 10   Calms tendons, eases pain in elbow, forelimb and sprains.

TH 14   Benefits shoulder problems, including lameness.

TH 17   Benefits all ear problems. Regulates estrous cycle.

TH 23   Aids all eye problems and eases pain.

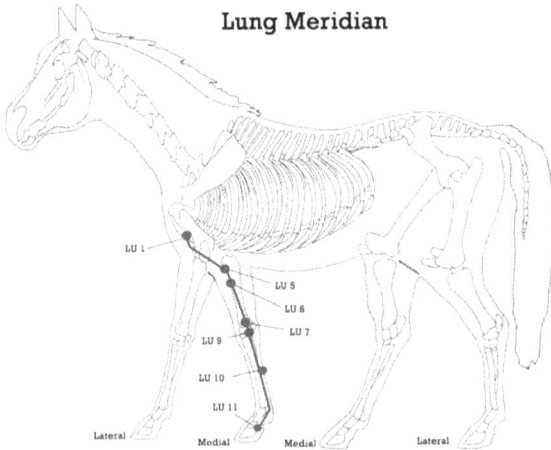

Lung Meridian

LU 1   Relieves respiratory problems
        and tones the lungs.

LU 5   Sedates excited conditions. Primary
        point for muscular and elbow disorders.

LU 7   Main point for the head, neck, and front
        limbs.

LU 9   Use for work with the arteries, to tone
        and clear respiratory problems and help
        with laminitis.

LU 11   Main point for acute respiratory
        disorders and nose bleeds. Boosts the

immune system and aids laminitis.

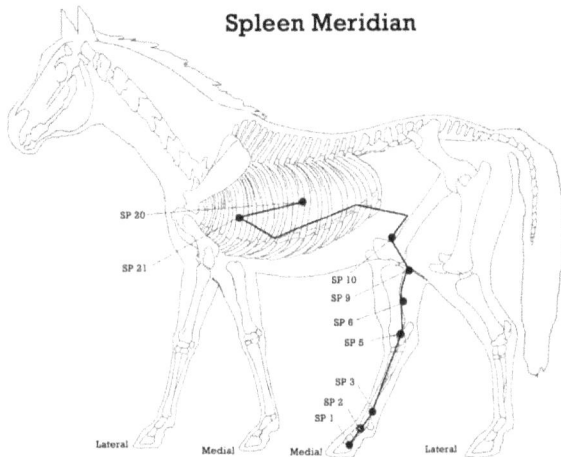

Spleen Meridian

SP 1   Balances energy and blood circulation.
        Aids the entire meridian, as well as
        laminitis and arthritis.

SP 2   Aids constipation and laminitis. Benefits
        the spleen.

SP 5   Strengthens connective tissues and
        eases stomach pain.

SP 6   Major junction of the spleen, kidney and
        liver meridians. Relieves fatigue,
        weakness, gastrointestinal and pelvic
        disorders. Boosts reproductive system in
        mares. Caution: May promote labor.

SP 9   Benefits the spleen. Aids stifle, urinary

and pelvic problems. Regulates the estrous cycle.

SP 10 Regulates the estrous cycle and boosts immunity. Helps pain in the stifle.

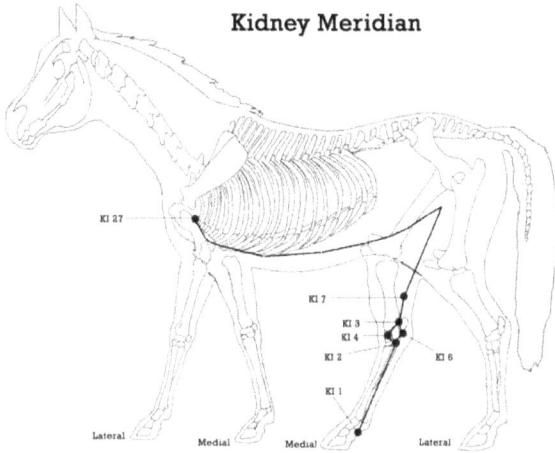

Kidney Meridian

KI 1   Eases shock and helps restore consciousness; treats laminitis

KI 2   Aids the pastern and tendonitis, also sexual dysfunction.

KI 3   Rebuilds immunity and regulates the estrous cycle. Aids hock arthritis.

KI 6   Regulates hormone production and releases hoof pain.

KI 7   Relieves fatigue, and hock and back pain.

KI 27   Main association point for every
         association point. Relieves respiratory
         problems and chest pain.

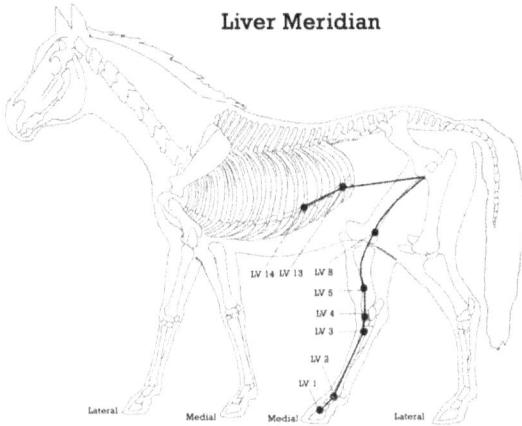

Liver Meridian

LV 1   Major point for laminitis or
        sidebone problems.

LV 2   Benefits colic and alleviates
        diarrhea.

LV 3   Clears and energizes the
        meridian. Calms and aids eyes.

LV 4   Helps lower abdomen, stomach
        and hooves.

LV 5   Regulates estrous cycles and aids
        hind leg soreness.

LV 8   Aids medial stifle conditions.

LV 14   Aids liver disorders and muscle soreness.

CHAPTER TEN

The Power of Purring:
A Case for Barn Cats

"For the want of a nail, the shoe was lost; for the want of a shoe the horse was lost; and for the want of a horse the rider was lost, being overtaken and slain by the enemy, all for the want of care about a horseshoe nail." ~ Benjamin Franklin

To date, cats have always been a welcome addition to any barn, keeping rodent populations in check and out of the feed. Now, there may be another reason to pamper your local barn cat, and encourage horse-cat relationships. Your friendly barn cat may just be the key to helping you or your horse heal faster.

The following research is excerpted from Elizabeth Von Muggenthaler's lay-paper, *The Felid Purr: A Healing Mechanism*. Von Muggenthaler is president of the Fauna Communications Research

Institute, a non-profit institute dedicated to the study of animal communication. The entire lay-paper, and more of the institute's groundbreaking research, can be found online at www.animalvoice.com.

All smaller felids, including the domestic cat, caracal, serval, puma, ocelot, and even some large cats such as lions and cheetah purr. A vocalization is used to display a particular emotion or physiological state. This enables an individual in society or pack to be able to express themselves. As any cat owner knows well, there are different "meows" for different emotions. This cannot be applied to the purr however. Cats purr even when they give birth and when severely injured in a barren cage at the veterinarian's. There are cases of cats purring when they are in grave physiological or psychological stress, as well as when they sit on your lap. Therefore, purring cannot be considered a vocalization, as the purr is produced under differing emotions or physiological states.

There is an old veterinary adage still repeated in veterinary schools that states, "If you put a cat and a bunch of broken bones in the same room, the bones will heal." Any veterinary orthopedic surgeon will tell you how relatively easy it is to mend broken cat bones compared with dog bones which take much more effort to fix, and take longer to heal. There is excellent documentation of the cats' quick recovery from such things as high-rise syndrome. First mentioned by Dr. Gordon Robinson in 1976, high-rise syndrome was later studied by Whitney, W., and Mehlhaff, C., (1987) in the Journal of the American Veterinary Medical Association. They documented 132 cases of cats plummeting many stories from high rise apartments, (average 5.5 stories) some suffering severe injuries. Interestingly, 90% of these cats survived. The record for survival from heights is 45 stories, however most cats suffer from falls of 7 stories or more and manage to live.

There has been some research that suggests that domestic cats are in general less prone to postoperative complications following elective surgeries. Using computer records, researchers state that complications following surgery for dogs undergoing castration to be averaged at 9.8%. The same surgery for cats lists the rate of complications to be 1.2%. Dogs undergoing *overiohysterectomies* (OHE) had complications 17.4% of the time and cats 8.4%.

Although it is impossible to standardize the healing time for dogs and cats in clinically occurring fractures, due to the type of fracture, amount of trauma to soft tissues, the type of treatment, the standard evaluation time or the after care, some general statements can be made. Cats do not have near the prevalence of orthopedic disease or ligament and muscle traumas as dogs do. Additionally, research suggests that non-union of fractures in cats is rare.

Dr. Clinton Rubin and his associates have made a fantastic discovery. They found that exposure to frequencies between 20-50 Hz (at low dB) creates the robust striations of increased bone density. In one study chickens were placed on a vibrating plate every day for 20 minutes, and grew stronger bone (*National Geographic, January 2001*, p. 11.) This discovery of anabolic frequencies between 20- 50 Hz (at low dB), is a tremendous breakthrough. Astronauts in space loose bone density in zero gravity, and this method could help them maintain healthy bones. This method is not yet FDA approved, although it is hoped it will be soon. Additionally, Zhonghua Wai Ke Za Zhi, in his work with rabbits, found that frequencies of 25 and 50 hertz promote bone strength by 20%, and stimulate both the healing of fractures, and the speed at which the fractures heal.

There is also documentation that low frequencies at low dB are helpful with regard to pain relief, and the healing of tendons and muscles. Vibrational stimulation between 50-150 Hz has been found to relieve suffering in 82% of persons suffering from acute and chronic pain. Biomechanical stimulation, which uses mechanical vibration of standardized frequencies from 18 - 35 Hz is used in Russian sports medicine. This technique improves the relaxation of strained muscle structures and increases the stretching ability of capsules and tendons. Lake in 1992, found that biomechanical stimulation prevents a decrease in muscle strength and muscle mass and the oxidative capacity of thigh muscles, following knee immobilization after sports injuries. The use of low frequency therapy also applies to tendon healing. It can increase the mobility of upper ankle joints by 16- 19 %. After ten days of short periods of biomechanical stimulation, upper mobility of ankle joints improved by 16 and 19 degrees and was accompanied by the healing of venous ulcerations after skin flap transplantation. It is interesting to note that Biomechanical stimulation is now also used in public gyms and work-out centers to increase muscle mass. A web search will bring up many manufacturers of such equipment.

We think that this research could help explain why cats purr, and here is why: Fauna Communications has recorded many cats' purrs, at a non-profit facility and the Cincinnati Zoo , including the cheetah, puma, serval, ocelot and the domestic house cat. After analysis of the data, we discovered that cat purrs create frequencies that fall directly in the range that is anabolic for bone growth.

* The dominant and fundamental frequency for three species of cats' purrs is exactly 25 Hz, or 50 Hz, the best frequencies for bone growth and fracture healing. All of the cats purrs fall well within the 20 - 50 Hz anabolic range, and extend up to 140 Hz.. All the cats, except the cheetah have a dominant or strong harmonic at 50 Hz.

* The harmonics of three cat species fall exactly on or within 2 points of 120 Hz which has been found to repair tendons. One species within 3 Hz and one within 7 Hz.

* Eighteen to thirty-five Hz is used in therapeutic biomechanical stimulation for joint mobility. Considering the small size of many of these cats, especially the domestic cats, it is interesting to note that all of the individual cats, have dominant frequencies within this range. Some of the cats have 2-3 harmonics in this range.

*   The frequencies for therapeutic pain relief are from 50-150 Hz. All of the individual cats have al least 5 sets of strong harmonics in this range.

*   Therapeutic frequencies for the generation of muscle strength lie between 2-100 Hz. All of the individual cats have al least 4 sets of strong harmonics in this range.

*   Therapy for COPD uses 100 Hz, all of the individual cats have a dominant frequency of exactly 100 Hz.

There is another clue found in a study performed by Dr. T. F. Cook. A dying cat who could not breath (they were considering euthanasia), was found to breath normally once it began purring. The purring opened up the cat's airway, and improvement was "remarkable and the next day commenced to eat...." Three species of cats have a strong harmonic at exactly 100 Hz, the vibrational frequency found to relieve dyspnea. One species within 2 Hz and one species within 7 Hz of 100 Hz. It could be that the cat's purr decreases the breathlessness by vibratory stimulation.

Is it possible that evolution has provided the felines of this world with a natural healing mechanism for bones and other organs? Researchers at Fauna Communications believe so.

Being able to produce frequencies that have been proven to improve healing time, strength and mobility could explain the purr's natural selection. In the wild when food is plentiful, the felids are relatively sedentary. They will spend a large portion of the day and night lounging in trees or on the ground. Consistent exercise is one of the greatest contributors to bone, muscle, and tendon and ligament strength. If a cat's exercise is sporadic it would be advantageous for them to stimulate bone growth while at rest. As well, following injury, immediate exercise can rebreak one and re-tear healing muscle and tendon. Inactivity decreases the strength of muscles. Therefore, having an internal vibrational therapeutic system to stimulate healing would be advantageous, and would also reduce edema and provide a measure of pain relief during the healing process.

It is suggested that purring be stimulated as much as possible when cats are ill or under duress. If purring is a healing mechanism, it may just help them to recover faster, and perhaps could even save their life.

(Excerpted with permission from Elizabeth Von Muggenthaler, *The Felid Purr: A Healing Mechanism*, Fauna Communications Research Institute, 2001)

Bibliography

Ausubel, K. *When Healing Becomes a Crime: The Amazing Story of the Hoxsey Cancer Clinics and the Return of Alternative Therapies.* Rochester, VT: Healing Arts Press, 2000.

Beston, H. *Herbs and the Earth: An Evocative Excursion into the Lore & Legend of Our Common Herbs.* David R. Godine, 1935.

Brennan, B. *Hands of Light : A Guide to Healing Through the Human Energy Field,* NY: Bantam, 1988.

Broken Bear Squier, T. *Herbal Folk Medicine: an A to Z guide.* Owl Books, Henry Holt & Co., 1997.

Carper, J. *Miracle Cures: Dramatic New Scientific Discoveries Revealing the Healing Powers of Herbs, Vitamins, and Other Natural Remedies.* HarperCollins Publishers, 1997.

Castleman, M. *Nature's Cures*. Rodale Press, 1996.

Cichoke Ph.D, A. *Secrets of Native American Herbal Remedies*. Avery, 2001.

Culpepper, N. *Culpepper's Complete Herbal*. W. London: Foulsham & Co.

Dobelis, I.N., Editor. *Magic and Medicine of Plants.* Pleasantville, NY: The Reader's Digest Assoc, 1990.

Duke, J.A. & Foster, *S. Peterson Field Guides: Eastern/Central Medicinal   Plants*, Boston: Houghton Mifflin Company, 1990.

Firebrace, P. & Hill, S. *Acupuncture: How It Works, How It Cures.* Keats Publishing, 1994.

Fischer-Rizzi, S. *The Complete Aromatherapy Handbook: Essential Oils for Radiant Health*. Sterling, 1991.

Fleischman, Dr. G. *Acupuncture: Everything You Ever Wanted to Know*. Station Hill Openings, 1998.

Gray, P. *The Organic Horse: The Natural Management of Horses Explained*. David & Charles, 2001.

Green, M. & Keville, K. *Aromatherapy: A Complete Guide to the Healing Art.* The Crossing Press, 1995.

Griffin Ph.D., J. *Mother Nature's Herbal.* Llewellyn Publications, 1997.

Harris, B.C. *Better Health with Culinary Herbs.* Barre Publishers, 1971.

Heinerman, Dr. J. *Natural Pet Cures: Dog & Cat Care the Natural Way.* Prentice Hall Press, 1998.

Hopman, E.E. *A Druid's Herbal.* Destiny Books, 1995.

Hutchens, A. *Indian Herbology of North America,* Boston: Shambhala, 1973

Hylton, W.H. & Kowalchik, C. *Rodale's Illustrated Encyclopedia of Herbs:*Rodale Press, 1987.

Kavasch, E.B. & K. Baar. *American Indian Healing Arts: Herbs, Rituals, and Remedies For Every Season of Life.* NY: Bantam. 1999.

Kavasch, E.B. *The Medicine Wheel Garden: Creating Sacred Space for Healing, Celebration, and Tranquility.* NY:Bantam Books, 2002.

Kavasch, E.B. *Native Harvests: American Indian Wild Foods Guide.* Expanded & Revised Edition. NY: Dover Publications, 2005.

Kavasch, E.B. *Native Harvests: American Indian Wild Foods & Recipes.* Expanded. Washington, CT: Institute for American Indian Studies, 1998.

Kidd, J.S. & Kidd, R.A. *Mother Nature's Pharmacy: Potent Medicines from Plants*. Facts On File, Inc., 1998

Macrae, J. *Therapeutic Touch: A Practical Guide,* NY: Alfred A. Knopf, 1987.

Maleskey, G. *Nature's Medicines*. Rodale Press, 1999.

Manniche, L. *An Ancient Egyptian Herbal*. British Museum Press, 1989.

Meeus, C. *Secrets of Shiatsu*. Dorling Kindersley, 2000.

Motz, Julie. *Hands of Life: From the Operating Room to Your Home, an Energy Healer Reveals the Secrets of Using Your Body's Own Energy Medicine.* NY: Bantam, 1998.

National Genetic Resources Program (NGRP). More than 80,000 plants in the data base.

http://www.ars.grin.gov/

Null Ph.D., G. *The Complete Encyclopedia of Natural Healing*.

Rand, W.L. *Reiki: The Healing Touch*. Vision Publications, 1998.

Restoring the Earth: Visionary Solutions from the Bioneers. Tiburon, CA: HJKramer, Inc, 1997.

Richardson, M.A., et al. "Flor*Essence herbal tonic use in North America: a profile of general consumers and cancer patients." *HerbalGram* 2000(50):40-46.

Roberts, Monty. *The Man Who Listens to Horses: The Story of a Real-Life Horse Whisperer.* NY: Random House; 1996.

Rose, J. *Herbs & Things*. The Berkeley Publishing Group, 1972.

Self, Hilary Page. *A Modern Horse Herbal*. Buckingham, UK: Kenilworth Press. 1996.

Schiller, C. & Schiller D. *500 Formulas for Aromatherapy: Mixing Essential Oils for Every Use*. Sterling Publishing, 1994.

Schnaubelt, K. *Medical Aromatherapy*. Frog Ltd., 1999.

Schoen, A.& Wynn, S.G.. *Complementary and Alternative Veterinary Medicine: Principles and practice.* NY: Mosby/Times Mirror. 1998.

Schoen, A. & Pam Proctor. *Love, Miracles, and Animal Healing: A Heartwarming look at the spiritual bond between animals and humans. NY:* A Fireside Book/ Simon & Schuster, Inc.. 1996.

Schoenbart L.Ac., B. *Chinese Healing Secrets*. Publications International, 1997.

Sigerist, H.E. *A History of Medicine*. Oxford University Press, 1951.

Stein, D. *Essential Reiki: A Complete Guide to an Ancient Healing Art*. The Crossing Press, 1995.

"The Ancient Herbal Tea that Became a Modern Cancer Tonic," in *The Doctors' Prescription for Healthy Living. Vol. 7 (8):* "Complementary Cancer Therapeutics." 2003.

Tierra, L. *The Herbs of Life: Health & Healing Using Western & Chinese Techniques*. The Crossing Press, 1992.

Wang, S.Y. and Zheng, W. **"Antioxidant Activity and Phenolic Compounds in Selected Herbs"**. <u>Journal of Agricultural and Food Chemistry</u>, **Vol. 49, No. 11: November, 2001.**

Worwood, V. *The Complete Book of Essential Oils and Aromatherapy*. New World Library, 1991.

Von Muggenthaler, E. *The Felid Purr: A Healing Mechanism*. Fauna Communications Research Institute, 2001.

A Medieval Herbal. Chronicle Books, 1994.

Botanical Names

Bilberry, *Vaccinium myrtillus*

Boneset, *Eupatorium perfoliatum*

Borage, *Borago officinalis*

Burdock, *Arctium lappa*

Calendula, *Calendula officinalis*

Celery, *Apium graveolens*

Chamomile, German, *Matricaria chamomilla*

Chaparral,_*Larrea tridentata*

Chaparral, Argentinean, *Larrea divaricata*

Chaste Tree, *Agnus castus*

Cleavers, *Galium aparine*

Clover, Red, *Trifolium pratense*

Comfrey, *Symphytum officinale*

Dandelion, *Taraxacum officinale*
Devil's Claw, *Harpagophytum radix*

Echinacea, *Echinacea angustifolia*

Elecampane, *Inula helenium*

Garlic, *Allium sativum*

Ginseng, Korean, *Panax ginseng*

Ginseng, American, *Panax quinquefolium*

Goldenrod, *Solidago Canadensis*

Hawthorn, *Crataegus oxyacantha*

Horsetail, *Equisetum arvense*

Kelp, *Fucus vesiculosis*

Licorice, *Glycyrrhiza glabra*

Marshmallow, *Althea officinalis*

Meadowsweet, *Spiroea Ulmaria*

Milk Thistle, *Silybum marianum*

Mullein, *Verbascum blattaria*

Nettle, Stinging, *Urtica dioica*

Oregon Grape, *Berberis nervosa*

Peppermint, *Mentha piperita*

Plantain, *Plantago major*

Prickly Ash, *Zanthoxylum americanum*

Raspberry, *Rubus idaeus*

Red Clover, *Trifolium pratense*

Sarsaparilla, *Smilax ornata*

Sheep Sorrel, *Rumex acetosella*

Slippery Elm, *Ulmus rubra*

Thyme, *Thymus vulgaris*

Turkish Rhubarb, *Rheum palmatum*

White Willow, *Salix alba*

Yarrow, *Achillea millefollium*

Index

B

C

About Earth Lodge

"Far back, far back in our dark soul the horse prances ... The horse, the horse! The symbol of surging potency and power of movement, of action ..." ~ D.H. Lawrence

The Birth of a Business

As modern New England "farmers/ gardeners" we've grown up with herbs and horses. We each come from generations of farming families, which inspires in us a deep appreciation and integrity for the land, animals, and healing. It seemed completely natural to develop a small business based upon these principals, incorporating the things we love best. It all began back in the 1990s with a unique educational concept, and grew to embrace larger practical aspects of herbalism, healing, and energy work. It has been a long and fascinating ride. (www.earthlodgebooks.com)

Author's Profiles

Maya Cointreau is a certified Reiki master in the Usui tradition, herbalism and a shamanic lightworker with over 20 years of experience. Herbalism is a continuing passion, and she is constantly reading new science reviews, books and journals to keep up with the "discoveries," as science sets about proving what folk herbalists have always known: Herbs work.

At Earth Lodge, Maya has spent the last 15 years formulating herbal remedies for animals, creating new flower essences, and providing hands-on healing therapies for people and animals alike. You can visit Earth Lodge on the internet at www.earthlodgebooks.com.

E. Barrie Kavasch is just a big flower fairy! She likes to write & draw plants.

Barrie is a botanical illustrator and master herbalist with a forty-year career in publishing books and articles for adults and young adults in both the popular trade and school and library fields. Her on-going success with *Native Harvests* led to *Enduring Harvests* (1995, Globe Pequot; 2002, iUniverse), plus the addition of select recipes in the award-winning anthology *EarthMaker's Lodge* (1995, Cobblestone), *American Indian Healing Arts* (1999, Bantam), and *The Medicine Wheel Garden* (2002, Bantam). She travels and lectures nationally and internationally, and has been guest lecturer on many college campuses and at numerous museums, environmental centers, and botanical gardens. The Herb Society of America gave her the "Gertrude B. Foster Award for *Lifetime Excellence in Herbal Literature*" in 2000.

Barrie founded the Medicine Wheel Wellness Center in CT, where she continues to teach and do energy work and shamanic healing. You can find out more about her range of work and many books at www.Kavasch.com.

Sandra Cointreau lives in two worlds.

Sandra is a environmental engineer with work in over 55 countries by day, and a world-class healer and President of IPLN, which produces Earth Lodge Herbals for Animals, by night. She has been studying various forms of healing for over 40 years, and is a certified Usui and Karuna Reiki Master, by William Rand, President, International Reiki Center.

She has also completed Healing Touch Level I with Carol Komitor of Healing Touch for Animals and Shamanism Level I with Michael Harner, President, Foundation for Shamanism Studies.

Sandra spent four years on daily intensive study of A Course in Miracles. She is a pleasure rider (hunter/jumper) and dog breeder (Stoney Brook Standard Poodles).

*"I don't mind what Congress does,
as long as they don't do it in the streets
and frighten the horses."* ~ Victor Hugo

More Books by Maya Cointreau

Practical Reiki Symbol Primer
The Comprehensive Vibrational Healing Guide
The Healing Properties of Flowers
Grounding and Clearing
The Girls Who Could Series
Equine Herbs & Healing
Natural Animal Healing
The Mudra Book

More Books By E. Barrie Kavasch

The Medicine Wheel Garden
Ancestral Threads
Hands of Time
Enduring Harvests
American Indian Healing Arts
Native Harvests
Earthwise
American Indian Earthsense
Guide to Eastern Mushrooms
Guide to Northeastern Wild Edibles
Introducing Eastern Wildflowers

More Books By Sandra Cointreau

Energy Healing for Animals

www.ingramcontent.com/pod-product-compliance
Lightning Source LLC
Chambersburg PA
CBHW072119270326
41931CB00010B/1608